Guide to Intellectual Disabilities

Julie P. Gentile · Allison E. Cowan
David W. Dixon
Editors

Guide to Intellectual Disabilities

A Clinical Handbook

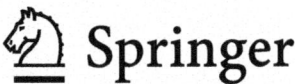 Springer

Editors
Julie P. Gentile
Department of Psychiatry
Wright State University
Dayton, OH
USA

Allison E. Cowan
Department of Psychiatry
Wright State University
Dayton, OH
USA

David W. Dixon
San Antonio Military Medical
Center
Houston, TX
USA

ISBN 978-3-030-04455-8   ISBN 978-3-030-04456-5   (eBook)
https://doi.org/10.1007/978-3-030-04456-5

Library of Congress Control Number: 2019931919

This Springer imprint is published by the registered company Springer Nature Switzerland AG
The registered company address is: Gewerbestrasse 11, 6330 Cham, Switzerland

For my amazing family, friends, and mentors; your enduring love, support, and guidance made this book possible. I love you all. Thank you!

~David W. Dixon DO

For my patients, from whom I have learned so much.
~Allison E. Cowan MD

To John Bertke and Patricia Gentile, my biggest fans.
To Sarah and Sayre, Jess and Jon, my biggest inspirations.
To Brynn, Harper, Wyatt, and Baby Byrd, my angels on earth.
To my patients, the strongest and most resilient individuals I've ever met.

~Julie P. Gentile MD

Contents

Contributors

Douglas K. Armour, MD Wright State University, Department of Psychiatry, Boonshoft School of Medicine, Dayton, OH, USA

Benjamin Lee Bates Registered Behavior Technician, S/OT, University of Findlay, Department of Occupational Therapy, Fairborn, OH, USA

Nita Bhatt, MD, MPH Department of Psychiatry, Wright State University, Dayton, OH, USA

Emily Bien, MD Department of Psychiatry, Wright Patterson Air Force Base, Wright State University, Dayton, OH, USA

Allison E. Cowan, MD Department of Psychiatry, Wright State University, Dayton, OH, USA

David W. Dixon, MD, DO San Antonio Military Medical Center, Houston, TX, USA

Julie P. Gentile, MD Department of Psychiatry, Wright State University, Dayton, OH, USA

Jeffrey Guina, MD Center for Forensic Psychiatry, Saline, MI, USA

University of Michigan Medicine, Ann Arbor, MI, USA

Department of Psychiatry, Wright State University, Boonshoft School of Medicine, Dayton, OH, USA

Kari Harper, MD Wright State Psychiatry, Boonshoft School of Medicine, Wright State University, Dayton, OH, USA

Ronne Justine Proch, DO, MA Wright State University, Boonshoft School of Medicine, Dayton, OH, USA

Wright-Patterson AFB, Department of Psychiatry, Dayton, OH, USA

Chapter 1
Introduction

Julie P. Gentile

A hero is an ordinary individual who finds the strength to persevere and endure in spite of overwhelming obstacles.

– Christopher Reeve

Approximately 2% of the population meets criteria for intellectual disability (ID), and these individuals will be encountered in virtually every clinical setting. There is a 3–6 times increased rate of psychiatric and behavior problems in individuals with ID compared to the general population. Progress has been made for the provision of high-quality medical and mental health treatment of individuals with co-occurring intellectual disability and mental illness. There remains a lack of universal training among most disciplines in this area, and stigmatization of both conditions continues to varying degrees. Current assessment and diagnostic classifications are available, including adapted criterion sets suitable for individuals with intellectual disability.

ID is categorized as profound/severe, moderate, or mild, which is often an indicator of the level of dependency needs and expressive language capability of the individual. The categorical designation is also frequently correlated with the level of risk for certain medical and neurological conditions.

J. P. Gentile (✉)
Department of Psychiatry, Wright State University,
Dayton, OH, USA
e-mail: julie.gentile@wright.edu

© Springer Nature Switzerland AG 2019   1
J. P. Gentile et al. (eds.), *Guide to Intellectual Disabilities*,
https://doi.org/10.1007/978-3-030-04456-5_1

Generally, individuals with *mild* cognitive deficits live independently in the community in supported residential situations with family or direct care professionals and participate in life-long supported employment. Special community-based vocational training is often required for success and to attain the highest quality of life. Persons in the *moderate* category will most often need varying levels of support from their families or community agencies. Because their expressive language skills are typically more limited, they are at a higher risk for inability to communicate subjective complaints about mental health and medical illnesses. Individuals with *severe/profound* ID are more likely to have very high levels of dependence on external supports and to have associated medical conditions, with most individuals requiring assistance for all aspects of life. Significant medical complications, such as seizure disorders, swallowing difficulties, speech impairments, ambulation limitations, sensory deficits, and reduced life expectancies, are more common for persons in the profound impairment category. Multiple physical disabilities increase the risk for medical complications irrespective of the level of ID.

It has been argued that the existing diagnostic manuals for mental disorders (i.e., *The American Psychiatric Association's Diagnostic and Statistical Manual for Mental Disorders*, Fifth Edition (DSM-5, 2013) [1], and *International Classification of Diseases* – Tenth Revision (ICD-10, 2014)) [3] may not fit well for individuals with ID. The Diagnostic Manual-Intellectual Disability, Second Edition (DM-ID-2, 2017) [2] is a manual that addresses the unique presentations of mental health conditions of individuals with ID. The manual takes into account decreased self-report and use of observational data; it is grounded in evidence-based principles and supported by expert consensus guidelines. The DM-ID-2 offers a review of scientific literature and research and, when appropriate, proposed alterations of diagnostic criterion for use in individuals with ID.

Patients with dual diagnosis often present to psychiatrists with behavioral change. Because these patients often have communication difficulties, they may have medical conditions which are undiagnosed and which affect their behavior. Characteristics of ID may confound the usual procedures for psychiatric assessment and treatment. The psychiatric interview of patients with ID can be complicated by communication deficits or lack of verbal communication skills, but by utilizing certain question types and avoiding others, one can yield a wealth of information as well as effectively develop rapport with the patient.

Most mental health (MH) care delivery systems have a different philosophy than most ID systems. For example, ID systems may meet the individual "where they are" without expecting significant change in functioning and focus on habilitation and self-determination, as opposed to MH systems which typically focus on "cure" and are recovery-oriented in that the expectation for mental illness is achievement of clear short-term goals. The ID professional relies on assessment of functioning while the MH professional relies on diagnosis. ID assessments view the entire person (living environment, employment, and medical), while MH assessments utilize the medical model to pursue diagnosis of disorders and underlying causes. The ID system offers involvement over the life span, holistic consideration of the person in the environment, and a detailed account of skills and behavior; the MH system offers crisis support, treatment of emotional distress, and behavior as a form of communication.

Patients with ID benefit from the full range of mental health interventions; however, there are important alterations necessary to ensure that mental health assessment, diagnosis, and treatment are effective and relevant. The use of the biopsychosocial formulation is the key to determining the etiology and true meaning of the behavior in the person with ID. Patients with ID often function at higher levels when accurately diagnosed, when psychotropic medications are prescribed following best practices, when medical conditions are appropriately treated, and when they have access to a full range of mental health treatments suitable to their developmental framework. Best practices and evidence-based medicine principles formulated for the general population are recommended when there are no unique guidelines available for individuals with ID. Overcoming communication barriers and connecting with an individual with ID is not only rewarding but should be the standard of care. Some say that individuals with ID are the most vulnerable in our society, but they are also the strongest and most resilient among us.

References

1. American Psychiatric Association, editor. Diagnostic and statistical manual of mental disorders. 5th ed. New York: American Psychiatric Association Publishing; 2013.
2. Barnhill J, Cooper S-A, Fletcher RJ. Diagnostic manual–intellectual disability 2 (DM-ID): a textbook of diagnosis of mental disorders in persons with intellectual disability. New York: National Association for the Dually Diagnosed Press; 2017.
3. http://www.ciproms.com/2012/08/examining-icd-10-cm-codes-for-mental-behavioral-and-neurodevelopmental-disorders-part-5/. Access date 06/01/2018.

Chapter 2
Psychiatric Assessment

Douglas K. Armour and Allison E. Cowan

The biopsychosocial model is the foundation of medical and psychiatric treatment. This model also gives greater understanding of the individual with intellectual and developmental disabilities. People with intellectual disability (ID) should be assessed in the same way that people without disabilities are: with care, compassion, and curiosity.

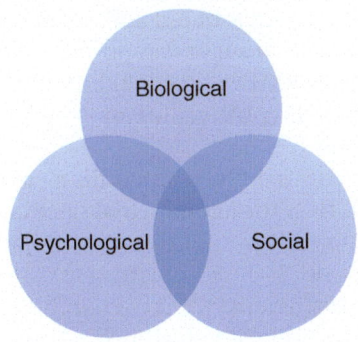

D. K. Armour
Wright State University, Department of Psychiatry,
Boonshoft School of Medicine, Dayton, OH, USA

A. E. Cowan (✉)
Department of Psychiatry, Wright State University,
Dayton, OH, USA
e-mail: Allison.cowan@wright.edu

© Springer Nature Switzerland AG 2019
J. P. Gentile et al. (eds.), *Guide to Intellectual Disabilities*,
https://doi.org/10.1007/978-3-030-04456-5_2

- *Biological Aspects*
  - Genetics: Obtaining a thorough family history is essential in determining the biological factors contributing to the presentation of a mental illness in a person with ID:
    - Many mental health disorders have a heritable component.
    - Family history of suicide increases risk of suicide.
    - Medical conditions including autoimmune disorders like lupus, thyroid disorders, or multiple sclerosis can present with primarily psychiatric symptoms and should be ruled out.
    - Specific genetic syndromes can carry associations with certain mental disorders, e.g., Fragile X and attention deficit hyperactivity disorder.
  - Non-psychiatric medical conditions can mimic or exacerbate mental illness:
    - For example, high blood sugar can cause irritability, while low blood sugar can produce panic-type symptoms. Anti-NMDA encephalitis can mimic schizophrenia. Hypothyroidism may present as depression.
    - Check routine labs including complete blood count (CBC) for anemia, leukopenia, and thrombocytopenia; comprehensive metabolic panel (CMP) for hepatic failure, electrolyte abnormalities, or renal insufficiency; thyroid-stimulating hormone (TSH) for thyroid dysfunction; glycohemoglobin-A1C for long-term blood sugar control; lead levels; and therapeutic medication levels.
  - Medication adherence:
    - Appropriate administration of prescribed psychiatric and non-psychiatric medications has a significant impact on the evaluation of an individual with ID.
    - Other medications may contribute to the individual's current presentation. New medications prescribed by other offices can have psychoactive properties, e.g., corticosteroids or interferon.

- Sleep status is an important part of mental health:
  - Untreated obstructive sleep apnea can cause irritability and aggression.
  - Disrupted sleep patterns can trigger manic episodes.
  - A good night's rest is essential for mental health.
- While less prevalent in persons with disabilities, the possibility of alcohol use or drugs of abuse should be considered.

- *Psychological Aspects*
  - Defense mechanisms:
    - Individuals with ID may be more prone to use developmentally "earlier" defenses.
    - Magical thinking is one of the most well-known earlier defenses in individuals with ID
    - Individuals with ID may use all levels of primitive, neurotic, or mature defenses.
    - Noting common uses of defenses in the ID population is important for assessment in relation to symptoms and level of functioning.
  - Temperament also plays a large part in presentation of psychiatric illness, and temperaments including slow to warm, easy, or difficult persist into adulthood.
  - An individual's attachment style impacts current relationships. Someone who experiences secure attachments as a child has an easier time with relationships as an adult; however, difficult attachment styles can also persist into adulthood.
  - Trauma can have long-lasting effects in building and maintaining relationships, can cause limitations in self-soothing during times of distress, and can impair an overall sense of feeling safe in the world.
  - Always assess for the possibility of current abuse as patients with ID are a vulnerable population.

- *Social Aspects*
  - Direct care professionals, mental health therapists, home health nurses, and habilitation specialists are important professional supports for individuals with disabilities and are also valuable collateral data sources.

- Financial security should be assessed as a contributing factor to mental illness. Inability to pay for food, medications, and outings can all impact the assessment.
- Access to resources including group psychotherapy or social skills classes, sensory/occupational therapy, applied behavioral analysis and support services, as well as individual psychotherapy should be determined.
- Habilitation/vocational services are an important part of recovery and stability as well as finding meaning and purpose in life.
- Friends, family, and romantic relationships are essential factors for optimal quality of life.
- Remember that individuals with ID may have large social networks, or they may have limited contact with family. Assessment of social involvement and supports is essential.

Practical Elements of a Comprehensive Evaluation of Individuals with ID

- Thoroughly review the available information from direct care professionals, behavioral assessments, other physicians, and the referral documents.
- Ensure that comorbid medical conditions are evaluated.
- These can include medication interactions or even conditions like cardiac abnormalities in young individuals as well.
- Coordinate care with the primary care physician to ensure good communication between providers.
- Establish routes of communication and collateral resources as individuals with ID often have unique means of communicating. Invested caregivers often can facilitate the flow of information between doctor and patient.
- The focus should be on the best interests of the patient and not necessarily what may make things easier for the treatment team.

Conceptual Issues to Keep in Mind with the ID Population

Table 2.1 describes the difficulties in interviewing individuals with ID (Table 2.1).

Managing the Interview

- Collateral information must be evaluated for clarity/relevance, clinical value, and accuracy.
  - An extensive pre-interview form with all relevant information is important:
    - This can include the chief complaint, history of present illness, family and social history, as well as other symptoms commonly encountered in the ID population such as seizures and genetic syndromes.

TABLE 2.1. Challenges in the diagnostic assessment of psychiatric disorders in people with intellectual disabilities

Cognitive disintegration	Vulnerability to decompensation under stress and subsequent overload of cognitive functioning may lead to bizarre, atypical, and even psychotic-like presentations
Psychosocial masking	Limited life experiences and intellectual capacity can influence the content of psychiatric symptoms
Intellectual distortion	Diminished abstract thinking and communication skills limit the ability of the person to accurately and fully describe emotional and behavioral symptoms
Baseline exaggeration	Pre-existing maladaptive behavior not attributed to a mental illness may increase in frequency or intensity with the onset of a psychiatric disorder

Adapted from Gentile and Gillig [1]

- The pre-interview documentation helps construct a conceptualization of the patient and guide the interview.
  - If the collateral information is not sufficient, it is appropriate to ask for a follow-up to be scheduled with staff who are able to provide further the information necessary for the evaluation.
- Identify the role designations of all present during an evaluation.
  - The role and familiarity with the patient are valuable as well as understanding who will be coordinating communication.
  - Understand that while the patient is your primary concern, the dynamics among other caregivers and the patient can lend valuable information.
  - A "difficult" patient will engender feelings in the people around them which can alter the efficacy of the care provided.
  - Understand that this population, while sometimes considered as being homogeneous, is in fact impressively heterogeneous. Each patient should be assessed as an individual and one must be careful not to jump to a diagnosis too quickly.
- Keep in mind that autism spectrum disorder has a wide variety of presentations and functioning levels.
  - Be aware of the body language of the patient. Individuals with ID and ASD often have limited capacity to cope with variations in stimuli and may display stereotypes and even have the inability to sit for an evaluation. Session flexibility is important and may help in certain cases.

Obtaining the History

- Always start evaluation by addressing the patient—even if it is as simple as having them express how they feel in the moment. The evaluation should start and end with the patient.

- Be mindful of the communication barriers faced by individuals with ID and that their answers may take longer to formulate than other patient populations. Patience is key:
  - Use simple vocabulary and avoid complex sentence structures.
  - Start with very concrete concepts like food or other basic needs and workshop/daytime habilitation activities and build from there. See Chap. 6 for additional information.
- Sequencing chronological events is often a struggle for the patient, but asking for caregivers to help frame reported events can be helpful.
- Limitations of attention, physical impairments including bowel/bladder incontinence, and even pain may limit an extensive interview.
- "Problem behaviors" may in fact be a physical malady that needs to be addressed such as hyperglycemia leading to frequent urination, which can be interpreted as the patient being "attention-seeking" as opposed to a physical need.
- Various screening/semi-structured interview tools can be used to help guide and provide an additional framework to the interview and should be used on a case-by-case basis.

Mental Status Examination: Modifications and Interpretations for Persons with ID

- *Observation:* It is important to use observational skills, especially as the capacity to communicate decreases. Ensure to note grooming, body habitus, and even cooperation with simple grooming tasks in which they receive assistance. Loud speech may indicate hearing impairment.
- *Orientation:* Determine the baseline orientation of the patient including orientation to person, place, time, and situation. Fund of knowledge is often limited due to intellectual disability.
- *Mood and affect:* Patients with less severe cognitive deficits are usually able to report their feelings and other

internal experiences of mood. It is often helpful to use simple vocabulary and/or visual displays, but understand that in the severely impaired, even simple vocabulary and pictures may not be adequate for a self-reported mood. Be aware of maturational age as this can also influence their mood/affect.

- *Thought disorder:* The psychotic symptoms reported by persons with ID are less complex and often insufficient to constitute a diagnosis of schizophrenia using standard diagnostic criteria. Auditory hallucinations are more reliably detected but negative symptoms are unlikely to be helpful in the differential diagnosis.
- *Cognition:* Excessive detail, rambling, and tangential thought process might represent the underlying cognitive impairments rather than a true thought disorder.
- *Risk of harm:* It is complicated by the limits or understanding of the potential lethality of a stated plan. They may repeat a phrase and may not even understand the precise content. It is important to have the patient describe as best they can the steps that are involved in their stated plan to assess intent, access, and opportunity.
- *Insight and judgment:* Many individuals with ID have insight and communicate that they are unwell even if they are struggling with a psychotic disorder by saying things like "I can't think" or "I'm not right." Even if formal insight may be lacking, they are often receptive to communication of advice/opinions of trusted family members, housing staff, work supervisors, and others.

Diagnostic Studies

- It is important to be an advocate for patients with ID and as such providers should have a low threshold to order laboratory testing as there are often comorbid medical diagnoses that could impact behaviors:
  - Electrocardiogram, complete blood count, comprehensive metabolic function, thyroid function tests, B12/folate, urinalysis, lipid panel, and VDRL.

- It may be beneficial to order blood levels of medications; also EEG, CT, and MRI may also be considered on a case-by-case basis.
- Urine toxicology screen may also be very important and should not be ignored in this patient population.
• See Chap. 3 for more information on medical assessment.

Differential Diagnosis and Diagnostic Overshadowing

• Differential diagnosis starts with attempting to clarify if one is faced with an underlying well-defined psychiatric illness like schizophrenia, depression, or anxiety/panic disorder or if what is being seen is more likely representative of the behavioral repertoire associated with the underlying ID.
• Diagnostic overshadowing is the process where health professionals are distracted by the disability itself and wrongly presume that the typical assessment and evaluation is not necessary. As a result, the patient receives inadequate diagnosis or treatment [2].

Stressful Life Events and Exaggeration of Baseline Symptoms

• Persons with ID have the same vulnerability to various life events as the general population and have been found to have more life events and transitions (moves, changes of job, new people in their lives) than people without ID.
• Social stressors can easily be overlooked if an individual with ID does not have the expressive language to communicate that they miss someone, that their best friend was not at the workshop today, or that they had an unfamiliar van driver. Being mindful of these changes can shed light on seemingly mysterious symptoms.

Conclusion

The psychiatric assessment of individuals with ID can outwardly appear different from an assessment of someone without ID, but the same underlying care is paid to the biopsychosocial model.

Clinical Pearls
- The biopsychosocial model gives an excellent framework to formulate the patient with ID.
- Remember that while patients can present with large treatment teams, the focus should be on what is best for the patient.
- Co-occurring medical conditions can mimic psychiatric illnesses.

References

1. Gentile, Julie P. and Paulette Marie Gillig. Psychiatry of intellectual disability: a practical manual. Hoboken:Wiley, 2012.
2. Reiss S, Levitan GW, Szyszko J. Emotional disturbance and mental retardation: diagnostic overshadowing. Am J Ment Defic. 1982;86:567–74.

Chapter 3
Medical Assessment

Julie P. Gentile and Emily Bien

Introduction

Recent studies have found that individuals with intellectual disability (ID) died 15 years younger when compared to the neurotypical population. The overall mortality for persons with ID is three times higher than for the general population. People with ID have higher rates of asthma and oral disease, and although epilepsy is one of the leading causes of premature death, there is little evidence on utilization of anticonvulsants to treat this specialized population [10]. More severe cognitive deficits and increased dependency on community supports are associated with shortened life span. Other risk factors associated with increased mortality include diagnosis of Down syndrome, inability to ambulate, deficits with motor skills, and self-help limitations [2]. See Table 3.1 for behavioral presentations in ID.

J. P. Gentile
Department of Psychiatry, Wright State University,
Dayton, OH, USA

E. Bien (✉)
Department of Psychiatry, Wright Patterson Air Force Base,
Wright State University, Dayton, OH, USA

© Springer Nature Switzerland AG 2019   15
J. P. Gentile et al. (eds.), *Guide to Intellectual Disabilities*,
https://doi.org/10.1007/978-3-030-04456-5_3

TABLE 3.1 Behavioral presentations commonly associated with medical conditions in patients with intellectual disabilities

Fist jammed in mouth	Gastroesophageal reflux disease, eruption of teeth, asthma, rumination, nausea, anxiety, painful hands/paresthesia, and gout
Biting side of hand	Sinus problems, eustachian tubes, ear problems, eruption of wisdom teeth, dental problems, pain, or paresthesia in hands
Whipping head forward	Atlantoaxial subluxation, other syndromes with joint laxity, dental problems, headaches
Intense rocking	Visceral pain, headache, depression, anxiety, medication side effects
Head banging	Depression, headache, dental problems, seizure, otitis, mastoiditis, sinus problems, tinea capitis
Waving head side to side	Attempts to supplement visual field, vertigo, hypervigilance, headache syndrome, vitreous humor
Walking on toes	Arthritis in hips or ankles or knees, tight heel cords
Won't sit	Akathisia, anxiety, depression, back pain, other pain, sleep deprivation
Sudden sitting down	Heart problems, syncope, orthostasis, medication side effects, vertigo, otitis, atlantoaxial instability, seizures, panic
Waving fingers in front of eyes	Migraine, corneal scarring, cataracts, seizures, glaucoma, diplopia, medication side effects
Wears multiple layers of clothing	Rule out endocrine and medication problems, post-institutional behavior
Covers eyes or ears	Consider psychosis, expression of hypersensitivity, preferences or fears, pain or depression
Places unusual wrappings on ankles, wrists, or other openings	Post-institutional coping, temperature regulation, or sensory integration issues
Glares with hostility at previously liked others or strangers	Rage or paranoia secondary to abuse or trauma history, psychosis
Wears costumes	Psychosis, expressing a wish or a fact from past or present

Brushes unseen material off body	Psychosis, dissociation, or neuropathy
Biting thumb or object with front teeth (or thumb sucking or bruxism)	Sinus problems, eustachian tube or other ear problems, finger pain, paresthesias, gout
Refuses to sit evenly or at all	Hip pain, low back pain, genital or rectal discomfort, ongoing abuse, clue to past abuse
Odd food refusals	*Odd food refusals* i.e., cravings or combinations, unusual aroma, family history of miscarriages, or dysmorphic features of developmental disability
Spells that are not generalized tonic clonic seizures	Most are related to anxiety disorders or tic disorders; however, if the usual treatment is not successful, consider testing for cardiac events or unusual metabolic conditions such as porphyria or G6PD deficiency
Intermittent fatigue	Multiple sclerosis, chronic viral infections, serum protein electrophoresis, lactate, pyruvate, comprehensive metabolic panel, glucose tolerance test, calcium, carnitine, B vitamins, iron levels
Ataxia	Atlantoaxial subluxation, heavy metals, fatigue
Joint swelling	ANA, rheumatoid factor, ESR, TB, syphilis screening
Partial seizures	B1, B2, B6, B12, folate, niacin, pantothenic acid, titanic acid
Snoring, history of airway obstruction, or history of brain injury	Sleep apnea, hypopnea, hypoxemia, or seizures
Flushing, rash, or other autonomic instabilities	Pheochromocytoma, carcinoid syndrome, porphyria, G6PD deficiency, autoimmune disorders, lyme disease, TB, syphilis, viral infections including HTV

Adapted from Ryan [15]

Diabetes Mellitus

- Adults with ID were significantly more likely to have diabetes than their counterparts in the general population.
- According to the American Diabetic Association (ADA 2010) [19], people with ID and others with specialized health-care needs frequently have nutrition concerns. These may include but are not limited to:
  - Growth alterations (i.e., failure to thrive, obesity, or growth retardation)
  - Metabolic disorders
  - Poor feeding skills
- Poor health habits, limited access to services, and long-term use of multiple medications are considered health risk factors, and these are frequently present in individuals with ID. Wilkinson et al. [21] propose that patients with ID may have risk factors which indicate that earlier and/or more frequent screening is essential for glucose monitoring.

Pulmonary System

Children with severe neurologic impairments have a higher incidence of respiratory problems. Common respiratory problems tend to be over-represented, especially in persons with cerebral palsy and/or traumatic brain injury. These conditions may secondarily lead to lung damage due to aspiration and ineffective cough.

- Patients are at an increased risk of morbidity and mortality of respiratory infections due to decreased airway clearance caused by muscular weakness and inadequate lung capacity.
- Conditions that adversely affect the lungs:
  - Drooling
  - Feeding problems
  - Gastroesophageal reflux
  - Aspiration

- Spasticity
- Scoliosis
- Gastroesophageal reflux and sialorrhea are associated with significant morbidity likely due to aspiration; appropriate medical care and compliance are vital to achieve improved quality of life [9].
- Regarding the pulmonary system, the Canadian consensus guidelines for primary health care of adults with developmental disabilities [18] state that it is vital to ensure vaccinations such as *Haemophilus influenzae* and *Streptococcus pneumoniae* are current. See Table 3.2 for screening tests for ID by organ system.

Gastrointestinal System

Children with neurodevelopmental disabilities such as cerebral palsy, spina bifida, or inborn errors of metabolism commonly experience gastrointestinal problems.

- Feeding difficulties, aspiration, and malnutrition are all potential consequences [17].
- Gastroesophageal reflux disease (GERD) is common in children with ID [9]. Researchers recommend a low threshold for the use of proton pump inhibitors [17].
- Constipation is a side effect of many medications including psychotropics, anticholinergics, and anticonvulsants, which result in fecal impactions. Van Timmeren et al. [20] reported a prevalence rate of more than 50% for people with severe and profound intellectual and motor disabilities.
- *Helicobacter pylori* (*H. pylori*) bacterium is an identified type I carcinogen that is correlated with peptic ulcers, gastric ulcers, gastric carcinoma, and primary B-cell lymphoma [6]. The prevalence of *H. pylori* infection in patients with ID is twice the rate of the general population; the recurrence of infection after triple-drug treatment is at a rate nearly seven times that of the general population. The Canadian consensus guidelines recommend the physician screen for *H. pylori* infection if there are persistent signs of

TABLE 3.2 Screening tests by system for individuals with intellectual disabilities

Diabetes mellitus	Sensory deficits
Screen for glucose monitoring early and more frequently Consult nutritionist for poor feeding skills, FTT, obesity, growth retardation, metabolic disorders	 Assess vision/ glaucoma once for age <40 (< 30 for DS) and then q2yr Assess hearing q5yr after age 45 (q3yr for DS) Screen for subclinical hearing impairment or undetected cochlear pathology

Pulmonary	Gastrointestinal
 Be careful of high risk of recurrent respiratory problems due to muscular weakness, ineffective cough, decreased airway clearance, inadequate lung capacity Risk factors: drooling, feeding problems, GERD, aspiration, spasticity, scoliosis Vaccinate for *H. influenzae* and *S. pneumoniae*	Be watchful for GERD, constipation (medical side effect), fecal impaction, aspiration, malnutrition, PICA, colonic volvulus and pseudo-obstruction (acute abdomen), reflux esophagitis (GIB) Risk factors: cerebral palsy, IQ <35, scoliosis, anticonvulsants, BZD, non-ambulatory

TABLE 3.2 (continued)

Menstruation	Cancer
Encourage regular GYN visits Be aware of mood/behavior changes plus abnormal bleeding Transdermal patch > OCP, Depo shot > IUD Side effects of anticonvulsants and antipsychotics can affect cycling and nutrition NSAID = pain, self-mutilation, aggression (caution for GI upset) SSRI = severe mood/physical symptoms in PMS/PMDD	Colon CA screening (early detection is difficult due to constipation) Prostate CA screening (same as general population) Breast CA screening (decreased parity and breast-feeding, physicians' lack of adherence) Cervical CA screening (based on sexual and FHx)

Adapted from: Wilkinson et al. [21]

dyspepsia or unexplained behavioral changes and to retest for *H. pylori* in 3–5 years after eradication of the bacteria.

- PICA: Khalid and Al-Salamah [5] reported that the general surgical problems related to the GI system necessitating admission in adult patients with ID included a history of PICA in 33% of cases.
- Volvulus of the colon (22.2%) and pseudo-obstruction (18.5%) were the most common causes of acute abdomen.
- GI bleeding: The most common cause (57.7%) was reflux esophagitis. Khalid (2006) [5] speculated that patients with ID not only experience these conditions at a higher prevalence, but also may have a higher threshold to pain when compared to the general population. To complicate matters, self-report is decreased due to communication difficulties. See Fig. 3.1 for various causes of GI symptoms.

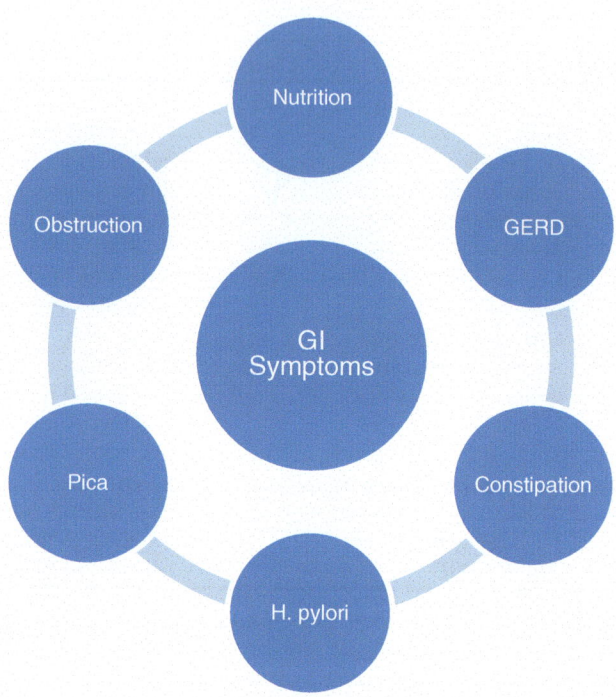

FIGURE 3.1 Various causes of GI symptoms

Menstrual-Related Conditions

- One of the most significant inequalities in medical care reported in the ID population is screening for breast and cervical cancer [3]. In this study, 11.5% of women with ID reported never having visited a and gynecologist; as a group they were significantly less likely to have undergone mammography. Despite the recommendation in the United States for women to have mammograms every 1–2 years beginning at age 40, 26.8% of the women with ID aged 40 and older in the Havercamp study had no documented mammography.

- Burke et al. [1] reported that girls with the diagnoses of Down syndrome, autism, and cerebral palsy presented for gynecologic treatment most frequently for menstruation problems (menorrhagia, dysmenorrhea, irregular bleeding, and hygiene issues) and mood/behavior changes. Medications frequently prescribed to patients with ID such as anticonvulsants and antipsychotics can affect cycle alterations. Bleeding abnormalities were the most prevalent complaints, and oral hormonal medications were the most commonly prescribed intervention:
  - Non-steroidal anti-inflammatory drugs (NSAIDs) should be considered a first-line treatment for cramping, pain and other [1] menstrual-related difficulties; use caution in patients who may be at risk for GI upset. Quint et al. (1999) [14] studied behavior problems in females with ID, including self-mutilation, aggression, and other behavior problems, and found that, with the use of NSAIDs, 65% showed improvement.
  - Oral contraceptives were effective in decreasing behavior issues in 40%. Depo-Provera injections were successful in treating 66% of the women in this study. Selective serotonin reuptake inhibitors (SSRIs) have been shown effective for severe mood and physical symptoms in premenstrual syndrome as well as premenstrual dysphoric disorder in placebo-controlled studies.

Cancer

Certain cancer types appear to be slightly more prevalent in adults with ID.

- Since constipation is a common problem for persons with ID, early detection of colon cancer symptoms may be difficult. The United States Task Force Guidelines for colon cancer screening should be followed without alteration for adults with ID.

- Breast cancer in women with ID was only slightly lower than that of the general population. Giving birth and a history of breast-feeding both have an impact on the prevalence rates. Women with ID are less likely to have children and to breast-feed; they are also less likely to undergo mammography due to the lack of physicians' adherence to preventive care recommendations.
- Cervical cancer is related to the number of sexual partners and frequency of sexual activity. Wilkinson et al. [21] ultimately recommend the decision be based on the woman's sexual and family history as opposed to her cognitive ability.
    - Fewer women with ID are sexually active, but there are other indications for periodic gynecologic examination:
        - Assessment for ovarian masses
        - Evaluation for fibroid tumors
        - Dysmenorrhea
- Prostate cancer screening was shown in two large studies to document lower rates of prostate cancer in men with ID compared to the general population. Wilkinson et al. [21] recommended that physicians screen their adult patients with ID as they would to other adults until more data is available.

Sensory Deficits

- Both vision and hearing problems can have a disproportionate prevalence and influence on adults with ID; sensory input is one compensatory mechanism to mitigate cognitive deficits. The Canadian consensus guidelines for primary health care of adults with ID [18] recommend referral of patients with ID for vision and glaucoma assessments at least once before age 40 (age 30 for patients with DS) and then every 2 years after age 40.

- High rates of hearing loss are reported in Turner syndrome, Down syndrome, Williams syndrome, and velocardiofacial syndrome (22q11 deletion syndrome).
- Mild hearing loss can have devastating costs even for typically developing children, specifically affecting vocabulary comprehension and syntax skills, receptive language skills, and development of attention and concentration patterns [8].
- The Canadian consensus guidelines for primary health care of adults with ID [18] recommend referring patients for hearing assessment every 5 years after age 45 (every 3 years throughout life for patients with DS). See Table 3.3 for syndrome-specific medical assessment. See Box 3.1 for clinical pearls.

Conclusion

Individuals with ID are at a significantly higher risk of having comorbid medical, genetic, and psychiatric conditions that in turn place them at a greater risk for medical conditions involving every organ system. Patients with ID are less likely to be afforded access to traditional preventative guidelines and treatment methods. The barriers to treatment must be overcome. It is well documented that neurotypical individuals with severe and chronic psychiatric illnesses have greatly reduced life expectancy; this is even more pronounced in persons with ID. Since many patients with communication deficits exhibit behavioral changes or acute psychiatric symptoms when experiencing medical conditions, the mental health clinician often plays a vital role in facilitating access to appropriate care.

TABLE 3.3 Medical conditions of common syndromes associated with intellectual disability by organ system

	Down syndrome	Fragile X syndrome	Prader-Willi syndrome	Williams syndrome
Classic Features	Broad short head, flattened face, epicanthal folds, flat nasal bridge, upward-slanting palpebral fissure, protruding tongue, small dysplastic ears, brushfield spots on iris	Long thin face, large protruding ears, prominent foreheads, facial asymmetry, wide head circumference, prominent jaw	Narrow bifrontal diameter, almond-shaped palpebral fissure, narrow nasal bridge, down-turned mouth	Short upturned nose, flat nasal bridge, long philtrum, wide mouth, full lips, widely spaced teeth, micrognathia, periorbital fullness, stellate iris pattern
General	No/lower fever than expected, premature aging	Early growth spurt, obesity, hypersensitive to stimuli	Obesity, hyperphagia, insatiable appetite, poor exercise tolerance, short stature	Overly friendly, hyperverbal, hyperactive, inattentive, poor weight gain, accelerated aging, early gray hair
Skin	Dry skin, decreased skin tone, recurrent skin infections, syringomas	Diffuse hyperpigmentation	Skin picking, hypopigmentation	Soft lax skin

HEENT	Atlantoaxial instability, cataracts, myopia/hyperopia, astigmatism, nasolacrimal duct stenosis, conjunctivitis, chronic otitis media, hearing loss, hypodontia,	Strabismus, nystagmus, astigmatism, ptosis, recurrent middle ear infections, dental overcrowding, high-arched palate	Strabismus, myopia	Esotropia, reduced binocular vision, hearing loss, hyperacusis, middle ear effusions, hoarse voice, increased interdental spacing
PULM	OSA, recurrent/chronic infections of URI/LRI, pneumonia	Pectus excavatum	OSA, cor pulmonale	Pulmonary stenosis
CARD	AV septal defect, tetralogy of Fallot, patent ductus arteriosus	Mitral valve prolapse	Right heart failure	Supravalvar aortic stenosis, mitral valve regurgitation, hypertension
GI	GERD, TE fistula, esophageal dysmotility, pyloric stenosis, duodenal atresia and stenosis, aganglionic megacolon, imperforate anus, diastasis recti, umbilical hernia, celiac disease	Inguinal hernias	GERD, aspiration, decreased ability to vomit, late cholecystitis, late appendicitis, gastric dilation	Inguinal and umbilical hernias, chronic abdominal pain, celiac disease
BACK	Scoliosis	Scoliosis	Scoliosis, kyphosis	Kyphoscoliosis, lordosis

(continued)

Table 3.3 (continued)

	Down syndrome	Fragile X syndrome	Prader-Willi syndrome	Williams syndrome
GU	Early menopause, hypogenitalism, hypospadias	Macroorchidism	Hypogonadotropic hypogonadism	Early menopause
MUS	Joint dislocation, joint hyperflexibility, flat feet, hypotonia	Joint laxity, flat feet, hallucal crease, small hands and feet	Neonatal hypotonia, arthritis, fractures, small hands and feet	Joint hyperelasticity, contractures, infant hypotonia, spasticity with age
ENDO	Annular pancreas, hypothyroidism (Hashimoto's thyroiditis), type 1 DM	Precocious puberty, premature ovarian insufficiency	Osteoporosis, hypopituitarism, ineffective thermoregulation, adrenal insufficiency	Hypothyroidism, hypercalcemia, hypercalciuria, slow weight gain, FTT, early puberty
HEME	Acute lymphoblastic leukemia, acute myeloid leukemia		Anemia from chronic rectal bleed 2/2 skin picking	
NEURO	Alzheimer disease, seizures	Seizures, stereotypic movement, tremor, ataxia	Cognitive impairment, stroke	Gross motor difficulties, hyperreflexia, nystagmus, visual-spatial difficulties

Decreased self-report and higher pain threshold

Adapted from: Jewell and Descartes [4], Lazier [7], Mundakel [12], Ng [13], Scheimann [16]

Box 3.1 Clinical Pearls

- Consider having patients weighed at home in a more familiar environment. The patients who are unstable when standing or have co-morbid physical disabilities may require a larger scale with more supports
- "White coat hypertension" might be more prevalent in people with ID. Portable electronic blood pressure may work well. Home monitors can measure the blood pressure in a relaxed familiar environment
- Blood draws may be best performed in familiar environments. For cholesterol and glucose testing, it is sometimes acceptable to use finger stick measurements. Studies have shown that finger stick measurement is acceptable for screening purposes especially in low- to moderate-risk patients younger than 65 years. However finger stick values can overestimate HDL and underestimate LDL so treatment decisions should ideally be based on venous samples
- Screen for cerumen is the first step in a hearing screening. Patients can then have a basic hearing test either in a primary care office or with an audiologist as needed
- Sedation may be required for routine procedures like dental work, endoscopic procedures, or minor surgery
- Menstrual-related psychopathology: Consult an OB-GYN to discuss regulation of menstrual periods. Consider conservative use of NSAIDs for menstrual-related changes
- If the patient has any chronic pain condition, rule out exacerbation at the onset of any problem behavior as well as a PCP exam and lab work-up.

Adapted from: McDermott et al. [11]

References

1. Burke LM, Kalpakjian CZ, Smith YR, Qunit EH. Gynecologic issues of adolescents with down syndrome, autism and cerebral palsy. J Pediatr Adolesc Gynecol. 2010;23:11–5.
2. Gentile JP, Monro M. Medical assessment. In: Gentile JP, Gillig PM, editors. Psychiatry of intellectual disability: a practical manual. Chichester: Wiley; 2012.. 26–50/51(abstract page). Print.
3. Havercamp SM, Scandlin D, Roth M. Health disparities among adults with developmental disabilities, adults with other disabilities, and adults not reporting disability in North Carolina. Public Health Rep. 2004;119:418–26.
4. Jewell JA, Descartes M. Fragile X syndrome. eMedicine. 2016. Retrieved 6/10/18 from https://emedicine.medscape.com/article943776-clinical#b4.
5. Khalid K, Al-Salamah SM. Spectrum of general surgical problems in the developmentally disabled adults. Saudi Med J. 2006;27(1):70–5.
6. Kitchens DH, Binkley CJ, Wallace DL, Darling D. Helicobacter pylori infection in people who are intellectually and developmentally disabled: a review. Spec Care Dentist. 2007;27(4):127–33.
7. Lazier J. Williams syndrome clinical presentation. eMedicine. 2015. Retrieved 6/10/2018 from https://emedicine.medscape.com/article/893149-clinical.
8. Marler JA, Sitcovsky JL, Mervis CB, Kistler DJ, Wightman FL. Auditory function and hearing loss in children and adults with Williams syndrome: cochlear impairment in individuals with otherwise normal hearing. Am J Med Genet C Semin Med Genet. 2010;154C:249–65.
9. Marks JH. Pulmonary care of children and adolescents with developmental disabilities. Pediatr Clin N Am. 2008;55:1299–314.
10. McCarthy J, O'Hara J. Ill-health and intellectual disabilities. Curr Opin Psychiatry. 2011;24(5):382–6. https://doi.org/10.1097/YCO.0b013e3283476b21.
11. McDermott S, Moran R, Platt T, Dasari S. Variation in health conditions among groups of adults with disabilities in primary care. J Community Health. 2006;31(3):147–59.
12. Mundakel GT. Down syndrome clinical presentation. eMedicine. 2018. Retrieved 6/10/2018 from https://emedicine.medscape.com/article/943216-clinical.

13. Ng N, Flygare Wallen E, Ahlstrom G. Mortality patterns and risk among older men and women with intellectual disability: a Swedish national retrospective cohort study. BMC Geriatr. 2017;17(1):269. https://doi.org/10.1186/s12877-017-0665-3.

14. Quint EH, Elkins TE, Sorg CA, Kope S. The treatment of cyclical behavioral changes in women with mental disabilities. J Pediatr Adolesc Gynecol. 1999;12:139–42.

15. Ryan R. Intensive conference on dual diagnosis. In: The community circle. Denver: CME Event; 2003.

16. Scheimann A. Prader-Willi syndrome clinical presentation. eMedicine. 2017. Retrieved 6/10/2018 from https://emedicine.medscape.com/article/947954-clinical#b1

17. Sullivan PB. Gastrointestinal disorders in children with neurodevelopmental disabilities. Dev Disabil Res Rev. 2008;14(2):128–36.

18. Sullivan WF, Heng J, Cameron D, Lunsky Y, Cheetham T, Hennen B, Bradley EA, Berg JM, Korossy M, Forster-Gibson C, Gitta M, Stavrakaki C, McCreary B, Swift I. Consensus guidelines for primary health care of adults with developmental disabilities. Can Fam Physician. 2006;52:1410–8.

19. Van Riper CL, Wallace LS, American Dietetic Association. Position of the American Diabetic Association: providing nutrition services for people with developmental disabilities and special health care needs. J Am Diet Assoc. 2010;110:296–307.

20. van Timmeren EA, van der Putten AA, van Schrojenstein Lantman-de Valk HM, van der Schans CP, Waninge A. Prevalence of reported physical health problems in people with severe and profound intellectual and motor disabilities: a cross-sectional study of medical records and care plans. J Intellect Disabil Res. 2016;60(11):1109–18. https://doi.org/10.1111/jir.12298.. Epub 2016 May 20.

21. Wilkinson JE, Culpepper L, Cerreto M. Screening tests for adults with intellectual disabilities. J Am Board Fam Med. 2007;20:399–407.

Chapter 4
Neurologic Conditions in Individuals with Intellectual Disability

Nita Bhatt and Jeffrey Guina

Seizure Disorders

Individuals with ID suffer from epilepsy up to 20 times more than the general population. For example, among those with cerebral palsy, about 30% have ID and, of those, about 40% have seizures. Additionally, Angelman syndrome, homocystinuria, Krabbes's disease, Lesch-Nyhan syndrome, Lennox-Gastaut syndrome, neurofibromatosis, phenylketonuria, Rett syndrome, Sturge-Weber syndrome, and tuberous sclerosis are also associated with both ID and seizures [8, 11]. The likelihood for seizures increases with the severity of ID and

N. Bhatt
Department of Psychiatry, Wright State University,
Dayton, OH, USA
e-mail: Nita.Bhatt@Wright.edu

J. Guina (✉)
Center for Forensic Psychiatry, Saline, MI, USA

University of Michigan Medicine, Ann Arbor, MI, USA

Department of Psychiatry, Wright State University, Boonshoft School of Medicine, Dayton, OH, USA
e-mail: guinaj@michigan.gov

© Springer Nature Switzerland AG 2019
J. P. Gentile et al. (eds.), *Guide to Intellectual Disabilities*,
https://doi.org/10.1007/978-3-030-04456-5_4

nearly one-half of individuals with severe ID suffer from seizures [5]. Up to one-third of individuals with ID do not develop seizures until adolescence or early adulthood [2]. Psychogenic non-epileptic seizures are more common in those with ID and epilepsy than the general population. Non-epileptic seizure-like activity may be due to transient ischemic attack (TIA), complicated migraine, syncope, hypoglycemia, narcolepsy, myoclonus, or conversion disorder. Of note, individuals with autism spectrum disorder (ASD) who do not suffer from seizures may show abnormal rhythms on electroencephalogram. Complex partial seizures are the most common seizures among patients with ID and ASD.

Dementia

A neurocognitive disorder—particularly a slow, progressive dementia—may be difficult to diagnose in those with ID due to overlapping symptoms, but it should be suspected if there is a decline from a previously obtained level. Many individuals with ID are at an increased risk for cognitive decline. For example, trisomy 21 is associated with early-onset Alzheimer's dementia—likely due to the amyloid precursor protein gene being located on chromosome 21—with up to 77% of individuals with Down syndrome developing Alzheimer's and up to 55% developing it before the age of 50 [7]. There is no cure for dementia, though lowering stroke risk factors (e.g., diabetes, hypertension, hyperlipidemia, smoking) may help prevent dementia, and acetylcholine esterase inhibitors and memantine may slow the rate of decline.

Delirium/Toxic Metabolic Encephalopathy

Individuals with ID—particularly severe ID—are at an increased risk of developing delirium [6]. Common underlying causes of delirium among those with ID are summarized in Table 4.1. Electroencephalography (EEG) often shows

TABLE 4.1 Common underlying causes of delirium in the ID population

Infection
Respiratory tract
Urinary tract
Medications
Anticholinergics
Antipsychotics
Anticonvulsants
Electrolyte imbalances
Dehydration
Fecal impaction

generalized slowing or, less commonly, abnormally fast activity [9]. Individuals with ID may experience hyper- or hypoactive delirium, though medication-induced delirium is rarely hyperactive [6]. Unfortunately, delirium in this population is more likely to go unrecognized, resulting in delayed treatment. Reasons for this may be misattributing cognitive or behavioral changes to ID and/or difficulty for those with ID to effectively communicate symptoms they experience. While ID and delirium may both involve disturbances in attention and cognition, a key distinction from ID is that delirium involves a disturbance in awareness (i.e., reduced orientation to the environment). Furthermore, these disturbances represent a change from baseline and tend to fluctuate in severity during the course of the day [1]. Patients with delirium are at an increased risk of falls, longer hospital stays, and increased cognitive decline and mortality rates during the year following hospitalization [12].

Delirium Case Vignette

Ms. A is a 53-year-old female with a past history of moderate ID, type 1 diabetes mellitus, and a TIA. She is brought to the hospital by group home staff for the acute onset of agitation and combativeness that has become progressively worse over the past 18 hours. A CT scan of the head was negative. Vital signs are within normal limits. Chest x-ray, urinalysis, and blood work are pending. While in the emergency department, the patient was noted to be agitated and frightened. She required soft restraints as she continuously attempted to leave her hospital bed despite staff and caretaker efforts to redirect and reassure her. The patient was admitted to the medical floor to evaluate the cause of delirium. A psychiatrist is consulted to assist with agitation, evaluates the patient, and meets with her mother, who is her legal guardian, to discuss treatment options. The psychiatrist recommends haloperidol injections as the patient continues to appear frightened and is combative toward caretakers and staff. However, the patient's mother is apprehensive about starting an antipsychotic, stating, "I hear those medications just sedate people in the hospital."

Treatment of Delirium

Definitive treatment of delirium requires identification of the underlying cause. However, this is not always immediately identifiable. Once the underlying cause is known, treatment involves reversing or addressing this underlying cause. Regardless of the cause, medications such as sedatives or anticholinergic medications should be discontinued or at least used with caution during the course of delirium.

Antipsychotics are the treatment of choice for agitation associated with delirium. It is important to explain to staff members and family members that the goal of treatment with antipsychotics in a delirious patient is not simply to sedate the patient but rather to prevent the individual from harming themselves or others. "As needed" antipsychotics should not be administered for convenience but rather for dangerousness. Haloperidol is the most commonly utilized agent when

TABLE 4.2 Environmental measures for delirium-related agitation

Orientation
  Place clocks and calendars in sight
  Open curtains during daylight
  Dim lights at night
  Frequently orient the patient to the time of day
Comfort
  Ask caregivers to bring treasured objects from home such as
  a favorite blanket or pictures of loved ones
  Encourage caregivers to visit frequently during the daytime
  Closely monitor and treat issues such as constipation or pain
Avoid over-stimulation
Minimize disruptions in nighttime sleep

managing hyperactive delirium. Acute delirium with agitation generally requires parental rather than oral antipsychotics, and haloperidol has both intravenous (IV) and intramuscular (IM) routes of administration. IV is preferable to IM haloperidol as it allows for more reliable absorption and, when an IV lock is present, may decrease the likelihood of causing distress to a delirious patient who might be confused or paranoid [12]. It is appropriate to monitor for QT prolongation with EKG or cardiac monitor and monitor vital signs and mental status regularly.

Environmental measures are also important for delirium-related agitation or "sundowning." Table 4.2 summarizes commonly used environmental measures.

Antipsychotic-Induced Movement Disorders

Individuals with ID are at an increased risk of developing medication-induced extrapyramidal symptoms due to their sensitive central nervous system [5]. The four common extrapyramidal adverse effects of antipsychotics include acute dystonia, akathisia, Parkinsonism, and tardive dyskinesia (see Table 4.3). The side effects may be treated by tapering and discontinuing the antipsychotic and switching to another agent

Table 4.3 Antipsychotic-induced extrapyramidal symptoms

	Characteristics	Onset	Treatment
Acute dystonia	Muscle spasm or stiffness (e.g., torticollis, trismus), tongue protrusions, oculogyric crisis	Usually occurs within the first hours or days of treatment and is most common in young males	Diphenhydramine, anticholinergics (e.g., benztropine, trihexyphenidyl)
Akathisia	Subjective feeling of restlessness and is in constant motion, unable to sit still, pacing, alternating sitting and standing	Usually occurs within the first few days of treatment. Most commonly occurs with the atypical antipsychotic Aripiprazole	Propranolol, benzodiazepines
Parkinsonism	Stiffness, cogwheel rigidity, shuffling gait, masklike facies, and is most common in elderly females	Usually occurs within the first few months of treatment, related to antipsychotic-induced dopamine depletion	Diphenhydramine, anticholinergics (e.g., benztropine, trihexyphenidyl)
Tardive dyskinesia	Perioral movements (darting or protruding movements of the tongue, chewing, grimacing, puckering), choreoathetosis of the head, limbs, trunk	Usually presents after years of treatment	Valbenazine, deutetrabenazine, some antipsychotics may suppress symptoms (e.g., quetiapine, clozapine)

(e.g., from a potent typical to an atypical antipsychotic). However, in some cases (e.g., comorbid psychotic or bipolar disorders, or ineffectiveness or worse adverse effects with other agents), continuing the antipsychotic and starting another agent to manage adverse effects may be appropriate.

ADHD

ADHD is three times more prevalent in children with ID, three to five times more common in children with comorbid ID and epilepsy, and more common among adults with ID [9]. Fetal alcohol syndrome, Fragile X syndrome, and DiGeorge syndrome are each associated with both ID and ADHD. The inattentive subtype of ADHD is more common in ID patients; however, those with the hyperactive/impulsive type have a worse prognosis and are more likely to suffer from conduct disorder or oppositional defiant disorder [9]. Mood dysregulation and aggression are common among those with comorbid ADHD and ID, and these individuals are more likely to be misdiagnosed with bipolar disorder [9]. Likewise, to ensure accuracy of ADHD diagnosis, it is important to assess individuals' schoolwork and activities in comparison to peers of similar developmental age (rather than chronological age). According to the DM-ID-2 [9], the ADHD diagnostic criteria adapted for persons with ID state that both inattentive and hyperactive/impulsive symptoms must persist to a degree that causes a direct negative impact and is inconsistent with the developmental level.

Treatment of ADHD

Stimulants including methylphenidate or amphetamines are considered first-line treatments for ADHD. Stimulants are generally well tolerated but adverse effects can include anorexia, nausea, insomnia, anxiety, irritability, and hallucinations. It is important to note that stimulants may induce or worsen tics; therefore caution should be used in individuals with comorbid ADHD and tic disorders. Common non-stimulant medications used in the treatment of ADHD include atomoxetine, bupropion, and alpha-2 agonists (i.e., clonidine, guanfacine). Behavioral interventions for ADHD include individualized education plans, psychotherapy, skills training, exercise, and parent education and training [3, 4, 10].

Tic Disorders

Tic disorders are common among those with ID [9]. Individuals with tic disorders display motor or vocal tics, which are sudden, rapid, recurrent, nonrhythmic, stereotyped motor movements or vocalizations. Tourette's disorder commonly presents with comorbid obsessive-compulsive disorder, ADHD, self-injurious behaviors, anxiety disorders, and depressive disorders [9]. The DM-ID-2 did not provide any adaptations for individuals with ID regarding Tourette's disorder, persistent (chronic) motor or vocal tic disorder, and provisional tic disorder. However, DSM-5 noted that "age of recognition and duration may be difficult to establish, especially if there are multiple genetic, neurodevelopmental, or medical conditions that may not be a direct contribution to tics (e.g. tics in individuals with Fragile X or trisomy 21)" [1].

Treatment of Tic Disorders

Atypical antipsychotics have been commonly used for the treatment of Tourette's disorder, though they have limited efficacy for common comorbid disorders such as ADHD and OCD. Alpha-2 agonists are effective in decreasing both the severity and frequency of tics and also treat ADHD.

References

1. American Psychiatric Association. Diagnostic and statistical manual of mental disorders. 5th ed. Washington, DC: American Psychiatric Association; 2013.

2. Boettger T, Rust MB, Maier H, Seidenbecher T, Schweizer M, Keating DJ, Faulhaber J, Ehmke H, Pfeffer C, Scheel O, Lemcke B, Horst J, Leuwer R, Pape HC, Volkl H, Hubner CA, Jentsch TJ. Loss of K-Cl co-transporter KCC3 causes deafness, neurodegeneration and reduced seizure threshold. EMBO J. 2003;22:5422–34.
3. Den Heijer AE, Groen Y, Tucha L, Fuermaier AB, Koerts J, Lange KW, Thome J, Tucha O. Sweat it out? The effects of physical exercise on cognition and behavior in children and adults with ADHD: a systematic literature review. J Neural Transm. 2016;124:3. https://doi.org/10.1007/s00702-016-1593-7.
4. Evans SW, Owens JS, Bunford N. Evidence-based psychosocial treatments for children and adolescents with attention-deficit/hyperactivity disorder. J Clin Child Adolescent Psychol. 2014;43(4):527–51.
5. Gentile JG, Gillig PM. Psychiatry of intellectual disability. A practical manual. West Sussex: Wiley; 2012.
6. Hassiotis A, Barron DA. Intellectual disability psychiatry: a practical handbook. West Sussex: Wiley; 2009.
7. Head E, Powell D, Gold BT, Schmitt FA. Alzheimer's disease in down syndrome. Eur J Neurodegener Dis. 2012;1(3):353–64.
8. Matthews T, Weston N, Baxter H, Felce D, Kerr M. A general practice-based prevalence study of epilepsy among adults with intellectual disabilities and of its association with psychiatric disorder, behaviour disturbance and carer stress. J Intellect Disabil Res. 2008;52:163–73.
9. National Association for the Dually Diagnosed. Diagnostic manual- intellectual disability: a textbook of mental disorders in persons with intellectual disability. 2nd ed. New York: National Association for the Dually Diagnosed; 2016.
10. National Collaborating Centre for Mental Health. Attention deficit hyperactivity disorder: diagnosis and management of ADHD in children, young people and adults. In: NICE clinical guidelines. Leicester: British Psychological Society; 2009.
11. Prasher VP, Kerr MP. Epilepsy and intellectual disabilities. New York: Springer; 2008.
12. Stern TA, Freudenreich O, Smith G, Fricchione G, Rosenbaum JF. Massachusetts general hospital handbook of general hospital psychiatry. Philadelphia: Elsevier; 2017.

Chapter 5
Traumatic Brain Injuries and Co-occurring Mental Illness

Emily Bien and Julie P. Gentile

Introduction

Assessment of the severity of TBI and the patient's cognitive, physical, and behavioral states early on is critical in establishing a treatment plan and tracking the progress of recovery. The Department of Defense and Department of Veterans Affairs classified the severity of TBI (see Table 5.1) based on Glasgow Coma Scores (GCS) (see Table 5.2), neuroimaging, and duration of loss of consciousness (LOC), alteration of consciousness (AOC), and post-traumatic amnesia (PTA).

Brain injuries can also be classified as primary or secondary. See Table 5.3 for TBI classification by type. Primary injuries are further specified as being focal, diffused, or mixed. Focal damage from direct impact tends to be visible on neuroimaging as a subdural/epidural hematoma, subarachnoid/intracerebral hemorrhage, or cortical contusion. Diffuse

E. Bien
Department of Psychiatry, Wright Patterson Air Force Base, Wright State University, Dayton, OH, USA

J. P. Gentile (✉)
Department of Psychiatry, Wright State University, Dayton, OH, USA
e-mail: julie.gentile@wright.edu

© Springer Nature Switzerland AG 2019   43
J. P. Gentile et al. (eds.), *Guide to Intellectual Disabilities*,
https://doi.org/10.1007/978-3-030-04456-5_5

TABLE 5.1 Classification of TBI by severity

Classification	GCS	Neuroimaging	LOC	AOC	PTA
Mild TBI	13–15	Normal	0–30 min	1 min to 24 h	0–1 day
Moderate TBI	9–12	± Abnormal	>30 min to <24 h	>24 h	>1 to <7 days
Severe TBI	3–8	± Abnormal	>24 h		>7 days

Adapted from Foley [3]. Department of Veterans Affairs (2010), page 11

TABLE 5.2 Glasgow Coma Scale

Eye-opening response (ER)	Verbal response (VR)	Motor response (MR)
4 = Spontaneous opening	5 = Normal	6 = Normal
3 = Opens to voice	4 = Confused but answers questions	5 = Localizes to pain
2 = Opens to pain	3 = Inappropriate responses	4 = Withdraws from pain
1 = No eye opening	2 = Incomprehensible speech	3 = Decorticate (arms flexed to the core)
	1 = No verbal response	2 = Decerebrate (extensor)
		1 = No motor response

Adapted from Glasgowcomascale.org [7]

TABLE 5.3 Classification of TBI by type

Primary injury	Secondary injury
Focal	Impaired cellular neurochemical cascade
Direct impact	
Often visible on neuroimaging	Impaired metabolic cascade
Diffuse	Increased intracranial pressure
Rotational force, acceleration, deceleration	Ischemia
	Hypotension
Less detectable on neuroimaging	Hypoxia
	Temperature dysregulation
Mixed	

Adapted from Foley [3]

injuries from rotational, acceleration, and deceleration forces are less detectable on neuroimaging. Secondary injuries have various etiologies, including but not limited to impaired cellular neurochemical and metabolic cascades, increased intracranial pressure, ischemia, hypotension, hypoxia, and temperature dysregulation.

Common Mental Health Presentations Following TBI/Co-occurring Mental Illness

Patients with TBI present differently based on the severity of the injury, their functional status prior to injury, location of injury, and type of injury. Depending on the location of injury to the brain, the patient may present with certain symptoms. See Fig. 5.1 for clinical presentation of TBI by anatomical location.

Traumatic brain injuries can affect some or every aspect of patients' health and present with varying combinations of cognitive, physical, and psychosocial symptoms. See Fig. 5.2 for symptoms of three domains affected by TBI.

Individuals with TBI may subsequently develop psychiatric illness. They may have mood disorders due to the injury itself or the resulting changes in their physical, emotional, and mental conditions. With regard to the central nervous system, a major depressive disorder in particular occurs more frequently after a TBI, compared to other psychiatric disorders. Within the first year of recovery, about 50% of patients with TBI will endorse depressed mood, anhedonia, and changes in sleep, concentration, appetite, or activity level [3].

Post-traumatic stress disorder (PTSD) symptoms will often manifest after patients suffer a TBI, which can further complicate the picture. Patients may have PTSD present several months after a TBI. Overlapping complaints of both PTSD and TBI would include depression, irritability, cognitive and attention deficits, difficulty sleeping, and tiredness. However, a thorough psychiatric assessment will reveal all relevant diagnoses. See Table 5.4 for a comparison of PTSD and TBI symptoms.

Psychotic disorders may also develop after a TBI. There is a possibility that patients who develop psychotic symptoms had increased vulnerability prior to the injury; however, the

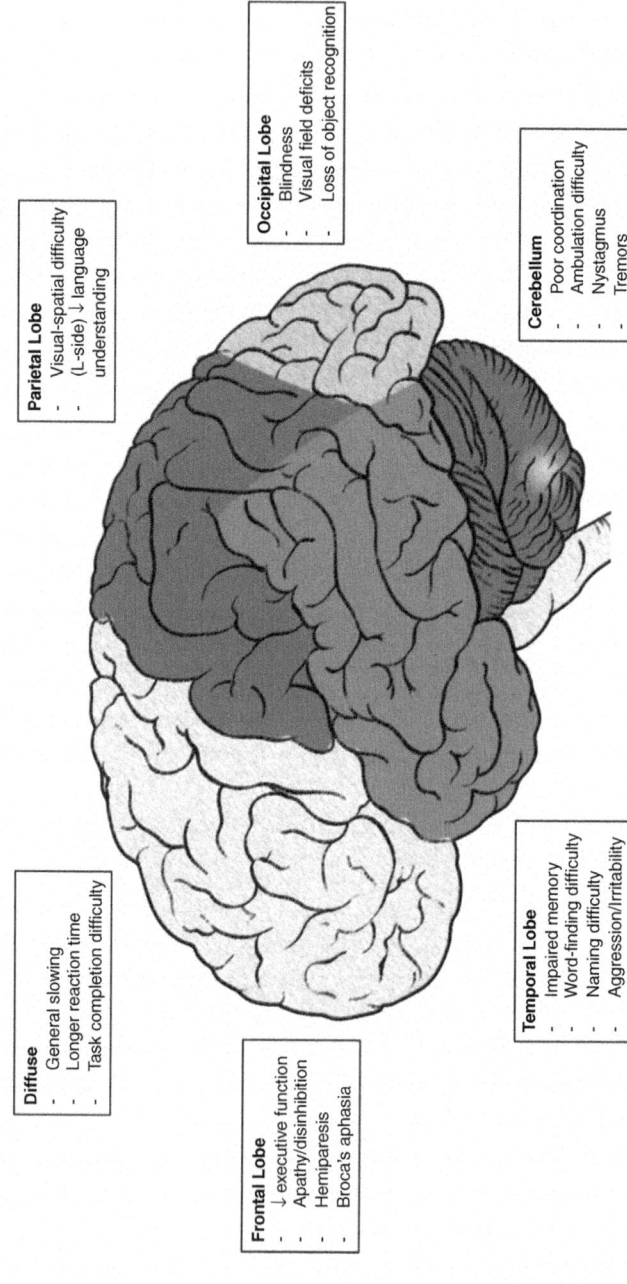

Parietal Lobe
- Visual-spatial difficulty
- (L-side) ↓ language understanding

Occipital Lobe
- Blindness
- Visual field deficits
- Loss of object recognition

Cerebellum
- Poor coordination
- Ambulation difficulty
- Nystagmus
- Tremors

Diffuse
- General slowing
- Longer reaction time
- Task completion difficulty

Frontal Lobe
- ↓ executive function
- Apathy/disinhibition
- Hemiparesis
- Broca's aphasia

Temporal Lobe
- Impaired memory
- Word-finding difficulty
- Naming difficulty
- Aggression/Irritability

FIGURE 5.1 Clinical presentation of TBI by location

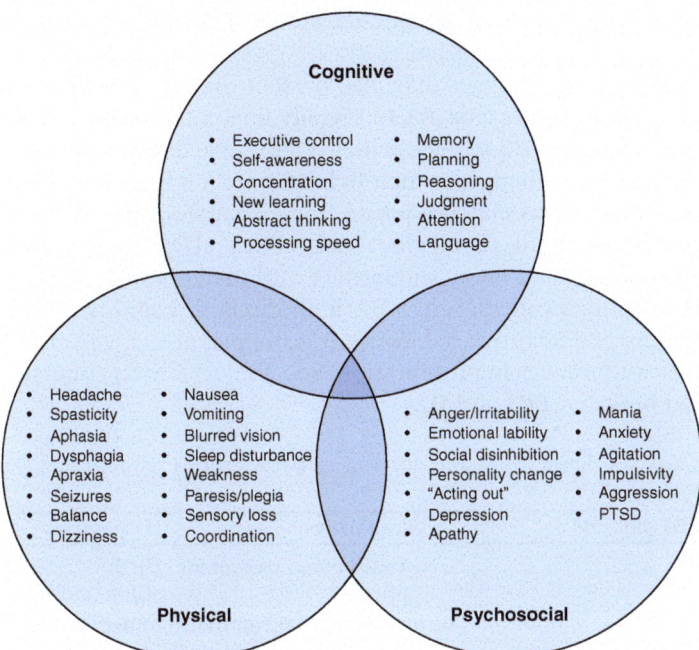

FIGURE 5.2 Symptoms of the three domains affected by TBI. (Adapted from Foley [3]. Department of Veterans Affairs (2010), pp. 6, 69)

TABLE 5.4 Similarities and differences between TBI and PTSD symptoms

TBI symptoms	Similarities	PTSD symptoms
Headaches	Difficulty in sleeping	Flashbacks
Nausea	Fatigue	Nightmares
Vomiting	Memory deficits	Avoidance
Visual changes	Inattentiveness	Hypervigilance
Light sensitivity	Anger/irritability	Intrusive recollections
Sound sensitivity	Depression/anxiety	Social isolation

Adapted from Foley [3]

strongest predictor was an identified first-degree relative with a psychotic disorder.

Personality changes may also present over time, which can range from subtle changes to socially unacceptable behaviors. Those who are close to the patients may have difficulty accepting that these changes in their behavior are not intentional and that the patients may not return to their previous baseline.

Patients with intellectual disabilities (ID) are another group that share many similarities with patients with TBI. As both groups can present with limitations in cognitive functioning and adaptive behaviors, it is important to be aware of their differences in presentation. See Table 5.5 for a comparison between TBI and ID.

TABLE 5.5 Similarities and differences between TBI patients and ID patients

TBI patients	Similarities	ID patients

Any age	Multifaceted treatment approach:
	  Med management
	  Non-pharmacological
	  intervention
		Birth/childhood up to age 22

Injury	Higher medication sensitivity:
	  Lower doses
	  Longer trials
	  Polypharmacy
		Genetic, congenital, injury, illness

Normal IQ
  Cognitive impairment
  Decreased attention
  Poorer concentration
  Impaired memory
  Delayed thought processing
  Difficulty with executive functioning and complex tasks
  Communication difficulties
	More comprehensive treatment:
	  Longer appointments
	  More frequent meetings
	ADL limitations
		Below-average IQ

Adapted from Foley [3]

Box 5.1 Clinical Pearls
- All providers involved in the patient's care should be aware of the multivariable presentation involving the physical, cognitive, emotional, and behavioral aspects after a TBI.
- Both patients with TBI and ID have higher medication sensitivity—start low and go slow; plan for lengthier medication trials.
- Obtain a thorough history of patient's baseline in all aspects prior to the TBI.
- Other diagnoses such as mood disorders, post-traumatic stress disorder, and intellectual disability may present with several overlapping symptoms with a TBI.
- Use extra caution with the use of antihistamines, narcotics, and benzodiazepines

Adapted from Foley [3]

Individuals who had a pre-TBI mental illness are at a greater risk of having persistent symptoms and may have more difficulty coping with the impairments resulting from the TBI. They may have decreased ability to develop adaptive compensatory behaviors, which limit their functionality and their recovery. See Box 5.1 for clinical pearls.

Clinical Vignette
Bystanders found a 26-year-old, unhelmeted, male unconscious after having lost control of his motorcycle. He was transported to the Emergency Department by an ambulance and was intubated. The physical exam revealed a GCS of 3 T and 3-mm bilaterally fixed pupils. A CT scan of the head showed a subarachnoid hemor-

rhage and left frontal subdural hemorrhage. He underwent a left-sided craniectomy and subsequently showed bilateral positive corneal reflexes and reactive pupils. Over the course of the next 2 weeks, his pulmonary function and GCS scores showed steady improvement. Psychiatry was consulted the following week due to "behavioral issues and non-compliance." He was started on low-dose sertraline, which improved mood and adherence and also decreased irritability. On hospital day 19, he was discharged to a nursing facility for long-term care and continued rehabilitation.

At a 6-month follow up, the patient was living with his mother. Residual deficits included motor aphasia and mood disorder. He required some assistance with daily living but could ambulate independently. Over the following 6-month period, his aphasia improved markedly with speech therapy, and his mood disorder was treated effectively with sertraline 150 mg daily. Despite a severe TBI and poor prognostic GCS scores/physical exam findings on initial assessment, this patient made significant gains in the first year of recovery. The importance of the multidisciplinary and interdisciplinary teams cannot be underestimated in the aftermath of a traumatic brain injury.

Treatment of Psychotic Disorder

Initially, a thorough history and physical examination should be obtained. This should include the patient's medical and psychiatric history, family history, social history including educational and occupational functioning, and substance use. A physical exam should include a mental status exam, mini-mental state exam, complete neurological exam, screening labs, and radiological imaging. Previous medical and psychiatric health records, educational records, and additional collateral information from family and friends should also be collected if possible. The Department of Veteran Affairs recommend asking specific questions in the initial interview to assist in development of a treatment plan. See Table 5.6 for recommended interview questions.

Depending on the severity and complexity of the patient's case, input from other specialties may be needed. Potential consults to be considered can be found in Table 5.7.

TABLE 5.6 Initial interview questions for patients with TBI

1. Why is the patient seeking evaluation at this time?	6. What is the global impact of the current symptoms?
2. What was the medical severity of the initial injury?	7. Is there a root cause to the current impairment?
3. What has been the recovery course since the event?	8. What is the patient's readiness to change?
4. What services/interventions have been utilized?	9. Are there other comorbidities to consider?
5. What are the severity/ duration of the symptoms?	10. How would disability status/ compensation affect care?

Adapted from Foley [3]. Department of Veterans Affairs (2010), pp. 2–4

TABLE 5.7 Possible consultants for patients with TBI as clinically indicated

Neurologist	Clinical psychologist	Physiatrist
Neuro-optometrist	Psychiatrist	Physical/occupational therapist
Neuro-ophthalmologist	Endocrinologist	Kinesiotherapist
Neurosurgeon	Audiologist	Recreation therapist
Neuropsychologist	Speech/language pathologist	Vocational rehabilitation counselor
Neurorehabilitationist	Social worker	Case manager

Adapted from Foley [3]. Department of Veterans Affairs (2010), p. 46

Management of Post-TBI Symptoms

Firstly, it is essential to assess symptom severity and cognitive changes early after a TBI. The management of mild TBI patients focuses on symptomatic treatment and cognitive rest, with a gradual return to baseline activities. For patients with moderate-to-severe TBI, short-term management will likely involve intensive care unit admission with consultations to neurology, psychology, and physical/occupational/speech therapy as clinically indicated and use of mannitol for reversing acute brain swelling and probiotics to decrease infection rate and length of hospital stay. Long-term management involves continued rehabilitation and monitoring of the progression of cognitive, physical, behavioral, emotional, and psychological comorbidities [4]. Furthermore, these patients and their families may not be familiar with resources available in the community and from the government. Connecting them to social workers and case managers can increase their independence and improve the transition to life after a TBI. See Table 5.8 for medication management to be considered in TBI.

Recent Research

In 2018, the FDA approved the first blood test to detect mild-to-moderate TBI by measure of two proteins, UCH-L1 (ubiquitin C-terminal hydrolase L1) and GFAP (glial fibrillary acidic protein) [5]. GFAPs are released by the brain into the circulatory system after head injuries. Patients presenting to the emergency department with suspected mild TBI or concussion undergo a CT scan of the head to check for intracranial lesions. However more than 90% of the patients will have a negative CT scan. This blood test, which is available within 3–4 hours, can reliably predict the absence of intracranial lesions, which would decrease unnecessary imaging. In addition, the severity of the trauma generally correlates with the levels of the protein markers, which are detectable up to 1 week after the TBI. This new laboratory test holds the poten-

Table 5.8 Medication management of TBI-associated symptoms

Symptom	First line	Second line	Notes
Headache prophylaxis	SSRIs, valproate	TCAs, topiramate, beta blockers, calcium channel blockers, trazodone	Avoid antidepressants in those with comorbid mania
Tension-type headache	Acetaminophen	NSAIDs	Avoid narcotics
Migraine-type headache	Triptans	Daily prophylaxis	Avoid narcotics
Insomnia	Zolpidem	Trazodone	Avoid benzodiazepines
Nightmares	Prazosin	Trazodone	Encourage sleep hygiene, consider imagery rehearsal therapy, or CBT
Fatigue/drowsiness	Caffeine (moderate use)	Methylphenidate, modafinil, amantadine	Try sleep hygiene first, rule out underlying cause (pain, sleep apnea, etc.)
Dizziness	Meclizine, dimenhydrinate	Benzodiazepine (low dose)	Consider ENT referral
Nausea	Ondansetron, promethazine	Prochlorperazine, metoclopramide	Monitor for QT prolongation, EPS side effects
Depression	SSRIs, SNRIs	TCAs, MAOIs, stimulants	Avoid bupropion (seizure risk)
Mania	Valproate, quetiapine	Carbamazepine, lithium	Other atypicals can be used, balance risks, benefits, side effect profile
Pseudobulbar affect	SSRIs	Dextromethorphan/quinidine, amantadine	

(continued)

Table 5.8 (continued)

Symptom	First line	Second line	Notes
Anxiety/PTSD	SSRIs	Buspirone, benzodiazepine (moderate half-life: lorazepam/oxazepam)	Avoid short-acting benzos (addiction potential, rebound anxiety) and long-acting benzos (cumulative side effects)
Psychosis	Antipsychotics (atypical)	Antipsychotics (typical)	Rule out delirium
Acute agitation	Antipsychotics (high potency)	Benzodiazepines	Rule out delirium
Disinhibited personality	SSRIs, anticonvulsants	Antipsychotics (atypical)	Avoid benzodiazepines
Apathetic personality	SSRIs, stimulants	Bromocriptine	Avoid benzodiazepines
Cognitive impairment	SSRIs, stimulants	TCAs, dopaminergic agents, donepezil, rivastigmine	Limit polypharmacy, utilize cognitive rehabilitation

Adapted from Foley [3]. Department of Veterans Affairs (2010), pp. 145–148

tial to increase the accuracy of rapid diagnosis and intervention with TBI.

Multiple studies have looked into the relationship between TBI and Alzheimer's disease, but results have been inconclusive and conflicting. However, recently two major articles have been published that have found an association between TBI and dementia. In 2018, data from the National Alzheimer's Coordinating Center were collected from 2133 participants with autopsy-confirmed AD and categorized by the presence or absence of self-reported TBI with LOC [6]. Those who sustained TBI with LOC greater than 5 min were found to be diagnosed with dementia about 2.5 years earlier than those who did not have TBI. Also in 2018, a nation-wide observational study was conducted using Denmark's comprehensive registry covering 2.8 million people with 132,000 episodes of recorded TBI over a 36-year period (1977–2013) [2]. It was found that those with a history of TBI had a 24% higher risk of dementia than those who did not have TBI.

Conclusion

Individuals with traumatic brain injuries can present with an array of symptoms that may appear over a course of time to varying degrees of impairment. A detailed, comprehensive data gathering of the patient's history and symptoms will result in an effective treatment plan. As with individuals with ID, patients with TBI will need a multifactorial approach in treating their various symptoms and co-occurring mental illnesses to improve the overall course of their recovery and functioning in all aspects of their life.

References

1. CDC.gov/traumaticbraininjury/data/statistics/index/html. Centers for Disease Control and Prevention. Traumatic brain injury and concussion. TBI data and statistics. 2013. Access date 17 May 2018.

2. Fann JR, Ribe AR, Pederson HS, et al. Long-term risk of dementia among people with traumatic brain injury in Denmark: a population-based observational cohort study. Lancet Psychiatry. 2018;5(5):424–31.
3. Foley GN. Traumatic brain injuries and co-occurring mental Illness. In: Gentile JP, Gillig PM, editors. Psychiatry of intellectual disability: a practical manual. Chichester, UK: Wiley and Sons; 2012. 75–89/90(abstract page). Print.
4. Jones KB, Wilson B, Weedon D, Bilder D. Care of adults with intellectual and developmental disabilities: traumatic brain injury. FP Essent. 2015;439:31–41.
5. Papa L, Brophy GM, Welch RD, et al. Time course and diagnostic accuracy of glial and neuronal blood biomarkers GFAP and UCH-L1 in a large cohort of trauma patients with and without mild traumatic brain injury. JAMA Neurol. 2016;73(5):551–60.
6. Schaffert J, LoBue C, White H, et al. Traumatic brain injury history is associated with an earlier age of dementia onset in autopsy-confirmed Alzheimer's disease. Neuropsychology. 2018. https://doi.org/10.1037/neu0000423. [Epub ahead of print].
7. Glasgowcomascale.org. What is GCS – Glasgow coma scale. [online]. 2015. Available at: http://www.glasgowcomascale.org/what-is-gcs/ [Accessed 16 May 2015].

Chapter 6
Interviewing Techniques

Nita Bhatt

Levels of Intellectual Disability and Categories of Communicative Skills

When conducting a patient interview, it is crucial to understand the individuals' level of ID as well as their expressive language skills in order to communicate effectively. Communication based on the level of ID is summarized in Table 6.1. It is important to note that most individuals with ID have better receptive than they do expressive language skills.

TABLE 6.1 Levels and communication

Mild ID	Verbal
	Uses concrete terms
Moderate ID	Verbal
	May answer questions with monosyllabic or other short responses
Severe or profound ID	Significantly limited verbal communicative abilities

N. Bhatt (✉)
Department of Psychiatry, Wright State University,
Dayton, OH, USA
e-mail: Nita.Bhatt@Wright.edu

© Springer Nature Switzerland AG 2019
J. P. Gentile et al. (eds.), *Guide to Intellectual Disabilities*,
https://doi.org/10.1007/978-3-030-04456-5_6

TABLE 6.2 Categories of communicative skills

Category of communicative skills	Description
Preverbal	Does not have cognitive ability to understand words
	Typically have profound and multiple learning disabilities
	Can be assisted through the use of routines, tone of voice, repetition, context of situations, objects, and their own experience
Nonverbal	Has ability to understand words, but does not have the ability to express themselves using words
	Will use alternative means to communicate, e.g., use of signing or pictures
Verbal	Has a variety of skills for understanding language
	Has expressive capabilities and predominantly uses speech

Adapted from Hassiotis et al. [2]

Though they may have limited verbal skills, they typically still understand what is being said during the interview. Categories of communicative skills are outlined in Table 6.2.

Challenges in the Diagnostic Assessment of Psychiatric Disorders in Individuals with Intellectual Disability

There are four difficulties in interviewing and assessing an individual with ID that are related to developmental delay and/or cognitive limitations [3]. Table 6.3 outlines these diagnostic challenges. Individuals with ID may display behaviors typical of early development throughout their adult life. Among the general population, these difficulties would be considered typical in a young child but abnormal in an adult. Some of these behaviors may include self-talk, imaginary

TABLE 6.3 Diagnostic challenges

Difficulties	Definition	Example
Cognitive disintegration	Impaired ability to tolerate stress leading to anxiety-induced decompensation that can lead the individual to appear bizarre, psychotic, or somatic	Patient with ID who recently moved to a new group home starts reporting a new imaginary friend. This could be considered normal behavior for ID though it may be considered bizarre for an individual in the general population
Psychosocial masking	Limited life experiences, social skills, and intellectual capacity can influence the content of psychiatric symptoms. These symptoms may be easily missed because they might seem normal for a neurotypical individual in the general population	Manic patient with moderate ID who believes he has a girlfriend and is able to drive a car. Though driving a car and being in a relationship is common for an individual in the general population, this may be a delusion of grandeur for a patient with ID
Intellectual distortion	Diminished abstract thinking and communication skills limit the ability of the person to accurately and fully describe emotional and behavioral symptoms	Patient with ID may answer "Yes" when the clinician asks if they hear voices. The clinician was referring to auditory hallucinations, while the individual was referring to ordinary voices such as the physician's
Baseline exaggeration	Pre-existing maladaptive behavior not attributed to a mental illness may increase in frequency or intensity with the onset of a psychiatric disorder	Patient with ID with aggression at baseline which can be controlled with behavioral techniques suddenly presents with increased aggression during a manic episode

friends, and fantasy play. It is important to note that these behaviors may be within normal limits for the individual's level of development and may not necessitate treatment [4].

Building Rapport

It is widely accepted among those in the medical community that a strong therapeutic alliance is essential to patient care and can have an effect on patient satisfaction, quality of life, and treatment outcomes. As with treating patients in the general population, it is important for the physician and the individual with ID to work collaboratively. In order to make the patient feel comfortable, it is beneficial to begin the interview by asking general, non-threatening questions such as their favorite activities, foods, or about their work or living arrangements. This also allows the physician to assess the patient's communication skills in a non-threatening manner.

Clinical Pearls for Interviewing Individuals with Intellectual Disability
- Be respectful.
- Match questions and answers to the individual's level of expressive language.
- Ask permission to involve collateral data sources.
- Collect collateral information and manage the triangle (See Chap. 2).
- Know what to expect. When possible, review all available medical records prior to the evaluation.
- Use simple language.

- Concretize the abstract.
- Use alternative ways to communicate when necessary (e.g., pictures, drawings).
- Ask the individual to repeat something if you did not understand what was said.
- Take responsibility for miscommunication.
- Eliminate distractions and unnecessary noise/movements during the interview.
- Do not use slang or figurative speech.
- Allow more time and consider multiple meetings if needed.
- Recap and summarize what occurred during the evaluation.

Interviewing/Evaluation of the Nonverbal Patient and Nonverbal Communication Across All Patient Populations

Across all specialties, physicians are trained to rely heavily on verbal communication, making the evaluation of the nonverbal patient particularly challenging. However, 60–65% of all interpersonal communication among individuals in the general population is conveyed via nonverbal behaviors [5, 6]. Having a better understanding of nonverbal communication can improve a physician's understanding of all patients regardless of their expressive language ability. Table 6.4 includes examples of nonverbal behaviors as diagnostic criteria for common psychiatric disorders. Table 6.5 describes universal expressions of emotions.

TABLE 6.4 Examples of nonverbal behaviors as diagnostic criteria for common psychiatric disorders

Autism spectrum disorders	Marked impairment in eye-to-eye gaze, facial expression, body postures and gestures; stereotyped, repetitive motor mannerisms
Attention-deficit/ hyperactivity disorder	Does not appear to listen when spoken to; easily distractible; fidgeting; inability to remain seated or attend to conversation
Substance intoxication or withdrawal	Cannabis intoxication: Conjunctival injection Opiate intoxication: Miosis Opiate withdrawal: lacrimation, rhinorrhea, yawning
Major depressive disorder	Psychomotor agitation or retardation; restricted or blunted, dysphoric affect; tearfulness
Post-traumatic stress disorder	Hypervigilance; exaggerated startle response; restricted range of affect
Schizophrenia	Flat affect, poor eye contact, avolition (negative symptoms); disheveled appearance, unpredictable agitation, rigid or bizarre postures (grossly disorganized or catatonic behaviors)

Adapted from APA [7]

TABLE 6.5 Universal facial expressions of emotion [8, 9]

Surprise	Jaw drops
	Opening the mouth without tension
	Eyes open widely
	Raised brows
	Forehead wrinkles horizontally throughout
Fear	Lips tense, stretch, and drawback
	Eyes open with lower lid tense and upper lid raised
	Brows raised, drawn close together
	Forehead wrinkles horizontally in the center only
Disgust	Upper lip raises and nose wrinkles
	Lower eyelid moves upward
	Brows are lowered

(continued)

TABLE 6.5 (continued)

Anger	Lips tightly closed
	Eyelids tense
	Brows are lowered and drawn close together
	Wrinkling appears vertically between the brows
Happiness	Corners of lips draw upward and nasolabial folds become prominent
	Lower eyelid raises and wrinkles appear around eyes
Sadness	Lips tremble or corners draw downward
	Eyes may tear
	Inner brows raise and draw together

References

1. Knapp ML, Hall JA. Nonverbal communication in human interaction. 7th ed. Wadsworth: Cengage Learning; 2010.
2. Hassiotis A, Baron DA, Hall I. Intellectual disability psychiatry: a practical, United Kingdom, handbook: Wiley Publishing; 2009.
3. Sovner R. Limiting factors in the use of DSM-III criteria with mentally ill/mentally retarded persons. Psychopharmacol Bull. 1986;22(4):1055–9.
4. National Association for the Dually Diagnosed. Diagnostic manual-intellectual disability: a textbook of mental disorders in persons with intellectual disability. 2nd ed. New York: National Association for the Dually Diagnosed; 2016.
5. Burgoon JK, Guerrero LK, Floyd K. Nonverbal communication. Boston: Allyn and Bacon; 2009.
6. Foley GN, Gentile JP. Nonverbal communication in psychotherapy. Psychiatry. 2010;7(6):38–44.
7. American Psychiatric Association. Diagnostic and statistical manual of mental disorders. 5th ed. Washington, DC: American Psychiatric Association; 2013.
8. Ekman P, Friesen WV. Constants across cultures in the face and emotion. J Pers Soc Psychol. 1971;17(2):124–9.
9. Ekman P, Friesen WV. Unmasking the face. Englewood Cliffs: Prentice-Hall Inc; 1975.

Chapter 7
Mood Disorders

David W. Dixon

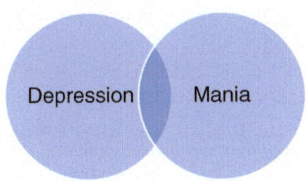

Depressive Disorders

Factors and Predisposition

- Depression appears to occur at higher rates among individuals with ID compared to the general population [1].
- People with ID are more likely to experience real and perceived losses throughout their lifetime like the loss of loved ones, pets, peers, roommates, or caregivers.
- The stress and grief from losses may predispose individuals with ID to more episodes of depression than the general population.
- Individuals with ID may also find that they often have diminished control in their lives with many activities and

D. W. Dixon (✉)
San Antonio Military Medical Center, Houston, TX, USA
e-mail: david.dixon@wright.edu

© Springer Nature Switzerland AG 2019
J. P. Gentile et al. (eds.), *Guide to Intellectual Disabilities*,
https://doi.org/10.1007/978-3-030-04456-5_7

life events dictated by caregivers, payees, guardians, and staff members, which can also contribute to depression.

- Personality structure can play a role in depression and is often exacerbated by feelings of rejection and internalization of negative interactions.
- Medical conditions in those with ID may be co-occurring, exacerbate, or mimic depression as well.
- Pain should always be considered with acute changes in behaviors or mood.

Evaluation

- *General Guidelines*: Ruling out medical conditions should be the first step to any evaluation of mental health issues [2].
- Individuals with ID may develop symptoms that look like depression from a wide array of medical problems including gastro-esophageal reflux disease (GERD), migraines, infections, medication side effects, or constipation.
- Sudden onset of severe symptoms warrants a thorough medical evaluation.
- Use developmentally appropriate language when directly questioning the patient (e.g., "Are you feeling sad?").
- For patients with limited verbal communication skills or limited cognitive abilities, use yes/no or closed-ended questions, and try to limit the use of open-ended questions to clarify specific points.
- Utilization of visual scales or inquiries about mood change (e.g., feelings of sadness) should be performed in conjunction with observation by the provider.
- Information from caregivers and family should be as objective as possible with specific behaviors identified and careful attention given to acute changes.
- Establish a clear picture of the patient's baseline. Discuss this at every visit to identify insidious changes not directly observable by staff with daily interaction.
- Psychosocial factors can have profound effects.

- Develop a timeline and the course of symptoms from caregivers if patients are unable to be specific.
- Ask about the time frame surrounding symptoms; try to identify any changes to routine, living conditions, social involvement, occupational changes, family members, stressors, or trauma.
  - Consider that any acute change following a stressor may be representative of a trauma- or stressor-related disorder.

Major Depressive Disorder

- Patients with ID may reach the threshold of clinically significant depression with fewer symptoms than required for the general population [3].
- Symptoms must be present for longer than 2 weeks.
- Depressed mood may be observed as no longer smiling or laughing, crying, flattened affect, or sadness.
- Irritability is commonly seen in lieu of, or in addition to, depressed mood and anhedonia. This may be observed as an angrier affect with agitation and has been included in the DM-ID-2 adaptation for major depressive disorder [4].
- Establish an understanding of patient sleeping patterns, habits, behaviors, and environment (e.g., bedtime, waking time, nocturnal waking, daytime naps, quality of sleep, nightmares/dreams, snoring, sounds in room, temperature fluctuations, type of bedding, roommates, etc.):
  - Rule out obstructive sleep apnea or other sleep disorders with a sleep study.
- Anhedonia may be observed as withdrawal from activities previously enjoyed, joyless participation, difficulty with motivation, and refusals or aggression with requests to participate in activities they previously enjoyed:
  - Clarify whether any changes to the activity have occurred like new participants or bullying which may result in behaviors that mimic anhedonia.

- Guilt/worthlessness may be observed as an increase in self-deprecating remarks, blame, or fears of punishment:
  - Those with severe to profound ID may not possess the cognitive ability to demonstrate feelings of guilt or worthlessness.
- Loss of energy may be observed as a change in typical functional level, amotivation, or subjective reports of being tired by the patient.
- Decreased concentration may be observed by changes in the ability to work or play, intermittent difficulties with memory, or difficulty completing common tasks.
- Appetite changes may be observed by refusal to eat favorite foods, weight loss/gain, and obsessing about or stealing food.
- Psychomotor changes may be observed by changes to typical behaviors, less sitting, agitated behaviors, or increase in verbalizations.
- Thoughts of death or suicide may be observed by increased talk of death or losses, talk of hurting themselves or others, increased focus on violence, or suicide attempts.
- Always evaluate for safety, especially regarding self-harm or harm to others. Establish intent, desire, plan, opportunity, and lethality.
- Involve caregivers and family in monitoring of changes in safety status and establishing safety plans.
- While atypical depressive symptoms may be more common with individuals with ID, pursue a thorough evaluation to rule out other causes and identify etiology (e.g., agitated irritability, visual hallucinations, olfactory hallucinations, mania, or hypomania).
- Individuals with ID may not fully meet criteria for depression; it is up to the provider to use their judgment to diagnose and treat, as they deem appropriate.

Persistent Depressive Disorder/Dysthymia

- People with ID with depressive symptoms present for more than 2 years have persistent depressive disorder/dysthymia [3].

- Evaluation should be treated the same as that with major depressive disorder, with a clear timeline important to determine whether asymptomatic periods exist.

Medication-/Substance-Induced Depression and Depression Due to Another Medical Condition

- Identify the medication, substance, or condition causing depressive symptoms.
- Identify a timeline of events to determine whether the depressive symptoms were present prior to exposure to presumed etiology.
- If a medication/substance is suspected to be causing depressive symptoms, determine next steps to address the issue.

Disruptive Mood Dysregulation Disorder (DMDD)

- Patients with ID may present with anger outbursts, irritability, and verbal or behavioral aggression well past childhood/adolescence [3].
- Consider the developmental age of the patient when determining whether a diagnosis may be appropriate.
- If DMDD is suspected, rule out any other disorders that could present with irritability.

Premenstrual Dysphoric Disorder

- Consider premenstrual dysphoric disorder when symptoms appear cyclical in nature and are correlated with the menstrual cycle [3]
- Tracking menstrual cycles for a person with ID is sometimes necessary to make this connection; consider the use of over the counter pain medication for physical symptoms

Treatment

General Considerations

- Discuss sleep hygiene and non-pharmacologic interventions; consider sleep study if indicated.

- Discuss dietary and exercise habits to improve overall well-being; consider consultation with nutritionist.
- When behavioral concerns are present, consult behavioral support specialists [2].
- Ensure individuals with ID are well integrated in the community (e.g., Special Olympics, charity events, sports leagues, church, art programs, community centers, libraries, etc.) to help improve self-esteem and social interaction.
- Consider music or art therapy consultation.
- Do not assume that individuals with ID are not sexually active and will not/cannot become pregnant.

Major Depressive Disorder/Dysthymia

- Treatment of depression in individuals with ID is not vastly different than treatment in the general population:
  - Mild to moderate episodes
    - Adapted psychotherapeutic interventions are effective.
  - Severe episodes
    - Antidepressants should be considered in conjunction with adapted psychotherapy [2].
- Adaptations to standard modalities improve efficacy in patients with limited expressive language or cognitive function. See Chap. 11 for more information.
- Antidepressant recommendations are based on best practices for the general population and are largely based on utilizing low doses, slow titrations, and single-medication changes with close observation.
- Medications should be chosen based on symptoms, comorbid conditions, and potential side effects, with careful consideration for adverse effects that may be more likely in people with ID.

Medication-/Substance-Induced Depression/ Depression Due to Another Medical Condition

- Treat the assumed underlying condition.

- If symptoms persist substantially (>1 month) beyond complete resolution of medical condition or substance/medication intoxication/withdrawal, consider reevaluating for depression or other comorbidities to guide further treatment.

Disruptive Mood Dysregulation Disorder

- Adapted interventions are the mainstay of treatment.
- Treat with antidepressants symptomatically with the same considerations given to major depressive disorder.

Premenstrual Dysphoric Disorder

- It is important that individuals with ID have access to preventive care; recommend consultation with obstetrician/ gynecologist or primary care physician to evaluate the menstrual cycle. Consider the use of over the counter pain medications for symptom relief.
- Antidepressant use may be beneficial; other treatment options may be preferable to minimize polypharmacy or to address the underlying etiology of symptoms.

Bipolar and Related Disorders

Factors and Predisposition

- The prevalence of bipolar disorder has been difficult to ascertain due to difficulty diagnosing the disorder based on standard criteria; it is likely similar to that of the general population.
- Patients with more severe ID are likely to be diagnosed with bipolar disorder (which may or may not be accurate),

likely owing to the fact that changes in baseline behavior are more likely to be reported by caregivers [1, 2].

Evaluation

General Guidelines

- Medical evaluation to rule out potential organic causes of depressive/manic/hypomanic symptoms (hypothyroidism, hypoglycemia, dementia, pain, medication side effects, substance withdrawal).
- Individuals with ID have higher rates of comorbid medical conditions.
- Pain can increase agitation, irritability, and create the appearance of a decreased need for sleep.
- Higher levels of communications deficits and lower developmental levels make evaluation of bipolar disorder especially difficult among those with severe to profound ID.

Mania/Hypomania/Major Depressive Episodes

- Rely on caregiver reports of activity-level changes when concern for mania/hypomania is present.
- Symptoms present at baseline may not indicate mania/hypomania.
- People with ID may present with fewer symptoms to meet the threshold of having mania/hypomania or depression.
- Major depressive episodes are evaluated in the same manner as major depressive disorder (see above).
- Manic and hypomanic episodes can be distinguished based on the length of time patient has the symptoms (hypomanic episodes will resolve prior to a week; manic episodes will not) or whether the symptoms rise to a level requiring hospitalization (hypomania does not typically require hospitalization).

- The key feature of any mania/hypomania will be that the patient presents with an increase in affective mood and energy.
- People with ID may be observed to be very silly, laughing inappropriately, intrusive, behaving in an expansive, excessive manner, or sometimes presenting as irritable (more common with severe to profound ID), demonstrating a departure from their baseline affect.
- Grandiose behaviors may be observed as the individual with ID claiming to be married to someone famous, having new abilities outside of reality, having a new job or task that is very important, or claiming to be a famous character or hero:
  - Distinguishing between developmentally appropriate wish fulfillment and magical thinking as opposed to psychotic symptoms is important and can be difficult even with caregiver input.
- Sleep disturbance may be a departure from usual sleeping habits with the patient getting less than 3 hours of sleep in a 24-hour period, without fatigue throughout the day, and no need for rest:
  - Often home staff will report that the patient is not sleeping when in fact there is napping throughout the day. This is more likely a sleep cycle disturbance rather than a bipolar symptom.
- Individuals with ID may have an increased amount of vocalization. Caregivers may report that the patient seems to talk endlessly about subjects with a distinct difference from their baseline conversation or that previous conversation topics appear to be more intense.
- Individuals with ID may switch topics rapidly, but those with mania/hypomania will demonstrate an increase in intensity or develop this type of thought process.
- Concentration difficulties (more common with depressive symptoms) and distractibility (more often related to mania) present very similarly.
- Mania/hypomania may also present with an increased sexual drive—including increased/inappropriate mastur-

bation—or increased drive to perform tasks. The person may move faster or be very active compared to baseline.

Bipolar Disorders (I, II, and Cyclothymia)

- Determining the difference between bipolar I disorder, bipolar II disorder, and cyclothymia is the same for individuals with ID and the general population.
- Identify a timeline of symptoms and determine if the patient has had symptoms consistent with mania/hypomania/depressive episodes now or in the past.
- The appropriate diagnosis will be based on whether mania has been present (bipolar I disorder), whether the patient has not had symptoms significant enough to be called mania/hypomania (cyclothymia), or whether the patient cycles between hypomania and depression (bipolar II disorder).

Substance-/Medication-Induced Bipolar and Related Disorder/Bipolar and Related Disorder Due to Another Medical Condition

- Attempt to identify the medication, substance, or condition that caused the symptoms and make appropriate intervention recommendations.

Treatment

General Considerations

- See recommendations for major depressive disorder (above).
- It is important to keep in mind that individuals with ID may often have multiple medications prescribed. Polypharmacy should be avoided and any psychotropic interventions should be carefully planned with the patient and caregivers.

- As in the general population, women of childbearing age should be informed of the risks of medications to any potential pregnancy even if family and caregivers think that the patient is not sexually active.

Bipolar Disorders (I, II, and Cyclothymia)

- There is limited research available addressing treatment of bipolar disorder in individuals with ID.
- Utilize appropriate evidence-based modalities for the treatment of bipolar disorder in the general population and apply these to people with ID.
- Valproic acid or lithium alone or in conjunction with second-generation antipsychotics for manic episodes is often effective.
- Valproic acid or lithium alone for hypomanic episodes may be helpful.
- Titrate to improvement of symptoms (just enough medications versus standard doses).
- The patient should be frequently evaluated for adverse effects, side effects, efficacy of treatment, response, or remission.
- See Chap. 10 for further details on mood-stabilizing and antipsychotic medications.
- Consider hospitalization if the patient cannot be provided with a safe environment or if presenting with mania.
- Involve family members and provide education about maintenance medications.
- Consider adapted psychotherapy to assist with depressive episodes and educate the team about this chronic medical condition.

Substance-/Medication-Induced Bipolar and Related Disorder/Bipolar and Related Disorder Due to Another Medical Condition

- Treat the underlying condition first [2].

- Consider treating manic episodes with valproic acid or lithium and/or second-generation antipsychotics as for bipolar disorder.
- If symptoms persist substantially (>1 month) beyond complete resolution of medical condition or substance/medication intoxication/withdrawal, consider reevaluating for depression, bipolar disorder, catatonia, or other comorbidities to guide further treatment [3].

Conclusion

- Medical conditions should always be ruled out before assuming the presence of a mood disorder.
- Individuals with ID suffer from depressive disorders at increased rates compared to the general population with no appreciable increase to the rates of bipolar disorders.
- Evaluating mood disorders requires the collaboration of patients and caregivers.

- Individuals with ID may present differently than the general population based on developmental level and cognitive/verbal/physical abilities.
- Thresholds for meeting criteria for mood disorder diagnoses may be lower than with the general population.
- Treatment options do not deviate significantly from those for people without ID.

Clinical Pearls

- Depression should be considered when an individual with ID is presenting with irritability or aggression.
- Mood disorders should be treated the same in people with ID as in people without.
- A multimodal approach with psychosocial interventions, medications, and behavioral interventions will support a patient in recovery from mental illness.
- Polypharmacy should be avoided.

References

1. Fletcher RJ, Barnhill J, Cooper SA. DM-ID-2: diagnostic manual-intellectual disability: a textbook of diagnosis of mental disorders in persons with intellectual disability. Kingston: National Assn for the Dually Diagnosed Press; 2016.
2. Gentile JP, Gillig PM, editors. Psychiatry of intellectual disability: a practical manual. Hoboken: Wiley; 2012.
3. American Psychiatric Association. Diagnostic and statistical manual of mental disorders (DSM-5®). Arlington: American Psychiatric Pub; 2013.
4. Fletcher RJ, Barnhill J, Cooper SA. Diagnostic manual – Intellectual disability. In: A textbook of diagnosis of mental disorders in persons with intellectual disability; 2016.

Chapter 8
Anxiety Disorders

David W. Dixon

Factors and Predisposition

- Patients with ID share similar biologic factors for developing anxiety disorders with general population [1]:
  - Dysregulation of the hypothalamic-pituitary axis
  - Dysfunction of neurotransmitter modulation
  - Antenatal stress
- Higher rates of anxiety disorders are seen among those suffering from specific genetic syndromes like Fragile X syndrome and Williams syndrome [1, 2].
- Individuals with ID may be more sensitive and susceptible to serious life events than the general population, with more anxious consequences stemming from such occurrences:
  - Transitions in workplace and home
  - Death or loss of caregivers and family
  - Serious medical illness
- Diagnostic overshadowing [3] is the process where health professionals attribute a symptom to the disability itself

D. W. Dixon (✉)
San Antonio Military Medical Center, Houston, TX, USA
e-mail: david.dixon@wright.edu

© Springer Nature Switzerland AG 2019   79
J. P. Gentile et al. (eds.), *Guide to Intellectual Disabilities*,
https://doi.org/10.1007/978-3-030-04456-5_8

and wrongly presume that the typical assessment and evaluation is not necessary:
- This is common in anxiety disorders.
- As a result, the patient can receive inadequate diagnosis or treatment.
• There can also be increased challenges to developing secure attachment in infancy and early childhood for people with ID.

Evaluation

General Guidelines

• Appropriate medical screening is the first step in evaluation of an anxiety disorder in intellectual disability [2, 4].
• Medical illnesses can cause symptoms consistent with anxiety which include but are not limited to [4]:
  - Hyperthyroidism
  - Myocardial infarction
  - Pulmonary embolus
  - Asthma
  - Infection
• Depending on the level of communication, it can be very difficult to assess anxiety levels in patients with more severe forms of ID.
• Observations from family and caregivers are crucial for evaluating any psychiatric diagnosis in the ID population but may be especially useful with anxiety [1, 4].
• Looking for changes in baseline is important. Identification of avoidant behavior, somatic complaints, sleep changes, obsessions, compulsions, excessive washing, rocking, difficulty sitting still, rumination with speech, mood changes, memory change, concentration change, increased fearfulness, agitation, crying, withdrawal, increased dependency, and an inability to sit still may all be signs of anxiety.
• Physiological signs may also be present, but the concern for an anxiety disorder should not cause a provider to

forego a medical evaluation. Some physiological signs of anxiety consist of dry mouth, flushing, sweating, tremor, headache, hyperventilation, diarrhea, increased urinary frequency, and insomnia.

- Establishing timeframes of symptoms can be challenging and will likely require the use of collateral information from caregivers or anchor events.
- Use developmentally appropriate language when directly questioning the patient (e.g., "Are you worried?" "Are you afraid?").
- For patients with limited verbal communication skills or limited cognitive abilities, use yes/no or closed-ended questions to screen. Limit the use of open-ended questions to clarify specific points or when talking with caregivers or family.
- Ask about the timeframe surrounding symptoms; try to identify any changes to routine, living conditions, social involvement, occupational changes, family members, stressors, or trauma [1, 4].
  - Consider that any acute change following a stressor may be representative of a trauma- or stressor-related disorder; see Chap. 15 for more information.

Generalized Anxiety Disorder

- Patients with ID suffering from GAD may not be able to report subjective symptoms, but caregivers should provide valuable objective information [1, 4].
- Individuals with ID may present with irritability, which may be externalized and observed as anger, agitation, or aggression toward others or property.
- The patient may describe an inability to control their worry about specific life events such as transitions, illness, or changes in caregivers; however, this may be dependent upon the severity of cognitive functioning.
- Caregivers may report that patient has insomnia or muscle tension.

- Establish a baseline for the patient's sleeping patterns, routines, behaviors, and environment [1, 4].
  - Details of bedtime, waking time, nocturnal waking, naps, quality of sleep, nightmares/dreams, or snoring can be helpful in elucidating patterns in sleep.
  - Consider the possibility of obstructive sleep apnea and the need for a sleep study.
- Decreased concentration may present as acute changes in the ability to work or play, intermittent difficulties with memory, or difficulty completing common tasks.
- The patient may exhibit anxiety by not being able to relax, pacing, or having a difficulty staying still, as well as other alterations from baseline behavior.

Panic Disorder/Panic Attacks

- A person with ID suffering from panic attacks may not be able to subjectively describe their experience, depending on their level of cognitive functioning [2].
- Patients with mild to moderate ID may be able to provide details regarding most of their symptoms.
- Many symptoms of panic attacks may be observed/reported by caregivers:
  - Cardiac changes are detectable with pulse or stethoscope.
  - Diaphoresis or tremor.
  - Extremes of hot/cold can be observed as flushing or shivering.
  - Shortness of breath sensation may be observed as hyperventilating or gasping for breath.
  - Feelings of choking may be observed with coughing.
  - Chest heaviness may be observed with clutching chest.
  - Nausea may be observed as dry heaves or vomiting.
  - Dizziness/lightheadedness may be observed with staggered gait, falls, or collapse.

Phobias/Social Anxiety Disorder/Agoraphobia/ Separation Anxiety Disorder

- Patients presenting with specific fears may not be able to describe their experience, though patients with mild to moderate ID are usually able to provide adequate information [1, 2].
- Evaluation may rely heavily upon observations from caregivers for severe to profound ID patients.
- Fear may be expressed behaviorally by tantrums, freezing, crying, and/or increased dependency.

Selective Mutism

- May present with refusal or inability to speak in certain situations but may be able to speak fluently in other situations that are familiar and comfortable.
- May not be able to provide insight into their condition, so diagnosis may require reliance on observations from others.
- Discuss with caregivers what situations and environments that the patient has demonstrated comfort with verbal responses.
- Utilize yes/no questions when interviewing the patient until an alliance is established to provide them with an opportunity to respond with signs and other non-verbal communication.
- Those with selective mutism may choose to whisper exclusively to one select person. That person can act as a liaison for communication until the condition improves.

Medication/Substance-Induced Anxiety/Anxiety Due to Another Medical Condition

- Attempt to identify the medication, substance, or condition that has caused anxiety symptoms.

- Discuss with patient and caregivers a clear timeline of events to determine whether the anxiety symptoms were present prior to exposure to presumed etiology.
- If a medication/substance is suspected to be causing anxiety symptoms, determine whether the substance is capable of causing the symptoms in intoxication/withdrawal or with regular use.

Treatment

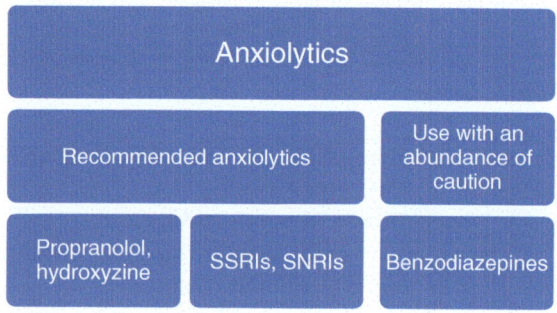

General Considerations

- Psychotherapy is a first-line treatment to help give the person a sense of agency and control over their symptoms [1, 4].
- The use of benzodiazepines in the ID population should be carefully monitored, and benzodiazepines must be used judiciously due to increased risk of disinhibition, worsened self-injurious behaviors, hyperactivity, or withdrawal-induced manic symptoms.
- When behavioral concerns are present, consult behavioral support specialists; see Chap. 12 for more information.
- Consider music or art therapy consultation.
- Do not assume that individuals with ID are not sexually active and will not/cannot become pregnant.

Generalized Anxiety Disorder (GAD)

- Psychotherapy and SSRIs should be considered first-line treatment [2].
- Treatment of anxiety in the ID population is not vastly different than treatment in the general population.
- A top-down (psychotherapy), bottom-up (antidepressant medication) approach is recommended.
- Psychotherapeutic interventions are effective but may require modification to address more severe deficits in expressive language skills and cognitive deficits.
- Individuals with ID can benefit greatly from psychotherapy with adaptations to accommodate memory and attention span difficulties [4].
- Antidepressant medications and specific anxiolytics (buspirone, propranolol) are appropriate for treatment of anxiety.
- Recommendations are based on best practices for the general population and are largely based on utilizing low doses, slow titrations, and single-medication changes with close observation [2, 4].
- Medications should be prescribed based on symptoms, comorbid conditions like hypothyroidism, attention deficit hyperactivity disorder, or cardiac disease as well as for potential side effects. Use extra caution. Careful monitoring in this population is recommended.
- See Chap. 10 for further details on antidepressant and anxiolytic medications.

Panic Disorder/Panic Attacks/Phobias/Social Anxiety Disorder/Agoraphobia/Separation Anxiety Disorder/Selective Mutism

- Adapted psychotherapy interventions are first-line treatments for these conditions [4].
- Cognitive behavior therapy, supportive therapy, exposure, and group therapy can be adapted to target specific symptoms, fears, or themes.

- Consider using an as-needed anxiolytic such as hydroxyzine for serious and disruptive panic episodes but not as a replacement for psychotherapy.
- Antidepressants or anxiolytics may be utilized with the consideration given to GAD (as above) but should be complementary to psychotherapeutic interventions [4].
- See Chap. 11 for more information on adapted psychotherapy.

Medication/Substance-Induced Anxiety/Anxiety Due to Another Medical Condition

- Treat the assumed underlying condition first [2].
- If symptoms persist substantially (>1 month) beyond complete resolution of medical condition or substance/medication intoxication/withdrawal, consider reevaluating for GAD or other comorbidities to guide further treatment.

Conclusion

- Persons with ID are susceptible to anxiety disorders.
- Evaluation of anxiety disorders in persons with ID requires some adaptations to classic criteria, involvement of family and caregivers, direct input from patients, and observations from providers.
- Limited ability to communicate can make it challenging to identify anxiety.
- Treatment options are similar to those available to the general population; however, they should be modified in order to better suit the needs of this specialized patient population.

Clinical Vignette

Mr. A is brought to his appointment because he is refusing to ride transportation to his day program. He has a kind and caring treatment team. Mr. A has habilitation staff who support him and look forward to seeing him each day. It is a source of confusion to his entire team that he has suddenly started refusing to attend his day program. He is brought to his psychiatrist for this inexplicable behavior. When asked, kindly and quietly, he shrugs and says that he does not know. No medication changes were made. Close follow-up was initiated and the following week, his roommate reported that the van driver had been abusive to Mr. A. The roommate herself was scared. The van driver was removed, but Mr. A continued to decline workshop. An SSRI was initiated along with psychotherapy for this traumatic event. Her team continued low-pressure encouragement to return to work, which Mr. A was able to do after about 1 month of treatment.

References

1. Fletcher RJ, Barnhill J, Cooper SA. DM-ID-2: diagnostic manual-intellectual disability: a textbook of diagnosis of mental disorders in persons with intellectual disability. Kingston: National Assn for the Dually Diagnosed Press; 2016.
2. American Psychiatric Association. Diagnostic and statistical manual of mental disorders (DSM-5®). Arlington: American Psychiatric Pub; 2013.
3. Reiss S, Levitan GW, Szyszko J. Emotional disturbance and mental retardation: diagnostic overshadowing. Am J Ment Defic. 1982;86(6):567–74.
4. Gentile JP, Gillig PM, editors. Psychiatry of intellectual disability: a practical manual. Hoboken: Wiley; 2012.

Chapter 9
Psychotic Disorders

Allison E. Cowan

Individuals with intellectual disability (ID) are estimated to have higher risk of developing a psychotic disorder than the general population [1, 2]. One proposed explanation for this increased rate is that often people with ID have higher rate of birth injuries, genetic disorders, seizures, and other factors that might make developing a psychotic disorder more likely. Diagnosis depends on the presence of the same symptoms as those in people with ID as those without a disability. A thorough history from the patient and collateral data sources is essential to accurate diagnosis and comprehensive treatment plan.

Diagnostic Criteria

Psychotic disorders are characterized by several core symptoms. These include hallucinations, which are defined as sensory experiences that do not exist outside the patient's experience, and delusions, which are fixed, false beliefs. In addition to these two symptoms, disorganized speech or

A. E. Cowan (✉)
Department of Psychiatry, Wright State University,
Dayton, OH, USA
e-mail: Allison.cowan@wright.edu

© Springer Nature Switzerland AG 2019
J. P. Gentile et al. (eds.), *Guide to Intellectual Disabilities*,
https://doi.org/10.1007/978-3-030-04456-5_9

thinking, disorganized behavior, and negative symptoms can be present in the diagnosis of psychotic disorders in varying combinations [3]. The Diagnostic Manual-Intellectual Disability, Second Edition (DM-ID-2) is a collaborative text from the National Association for the Dually Diagnosed (NADD) that has carefully adapted the diagnostic criteria for improved psychiatric diagnosis in individuals with ID.

Schizophrenia (from DM-ID-2)

DM-ID-2: *No adaptation for those with mild and moderate ID. Note for individuals with severe and profound ID: There may be self-talk which is common and not necessarily interpreted as an expression of psychotic disorder* [4]

- Psychotic symptoms in individuals with ID are similar to those experienced by people without ID and include hallucinations and delusions.
  - Hallucinations
    - Hallucinations are sensory experiences, typically auditory, that are experienced as real by the patient.
    - The most common types of hallucinations are hearing voices or whispers out loud. They can be heard saying indistinct or derogatory things to or about the patient. These hallucinations will typically be based in some fear or uncertainty that is correlated to a real and existing fear of the patient.
    - Typical hallucinations are voices that are scary to the patient. For example, an individual with ID may experience voices yelling that they have to move out of their cherished housing placement or that there are people coming to kill them. These are not dissimilar to people with schizophrenia that do not have ID.
  - Delusions
    - Delusions are fixed, false beliefs that are unable to be dissuaded with argument, logic, or proof to the contrary

- Typical delusions can include
  - Paranoid delusions—the belief that certain people or groups are targeting the patient specifically to harm them or to harm their loved ones
  - Grandiose delusions—the belief that the patient is a famous or influential person like Gandhi, Madonna, or Michael Jackson
  - Somatic delusions—that a body part has been stolen or is trying to kill them from the inside

DM-ID-2: *No adaptations for the criteria B-F for schizophrenia* [4]

- For a person to be diagnosed with a disorder, certain other signifiers of illness must be present. These are unchanged in people with ID when compared with individuals without ID.
- A person with ID who has schizophrenia might require more assistance with activities of daily living at baseline than someone without ID. This should be taken into account when making the diagnosis of schizophrenia.
- Additionally an individual with ID with supported or sheltered employment might have certain allowances in work performance that do not have direct consequences to their employment, but information should be gathered from habilitation and vocational contacts about work performance.

Schizoaffective Disorder

DM-ID-2: *No adaptations for Criteria A-D* [4]

- Schizoaffective disorder is a psychotic disorder that exists on a spectrum somewhere between, on the one end, an affective disorder like depression or bipolar disorder and, on the other, solely psychotic disorders like schizophrenia.
- In order to be diagnosed with schizoaffective disorder, the individual must experience psychotic symptoms that do not occur during a manic or depressive episode.

- Experts in the ID field suggest that no change in the diagnostic criteria be made for individuals with ID [4].
- Treatment for schizoaffective disorders remains the same as for those with ID as it is for the general population.
  - Medications that address psychotic and affective symptoms, such as second-generation antipsychotic medications approved for the treatment of both affective and psychotic symptoms are typically recommended as first line.
  - Polypharmacy may be required to treat psychotic symptoms as well as affective ones.
    - Depression that is part of schizoaffective disorder may be addressed with an antidepressant.
    - Mania may be treated with antimanic agents like valproic acid or lithium. See Chap. 11 for additional information.

Delusional Disorder

DM-ID-2: *No adaptation for those with Mild and Moderate ID. The criteria for diagnosis do not apply for those with Severe and Profound ID* [4]

- Delusional disorder is described as an individual having a single, discrete delusion without other symptoms of schizophrenia such as hallucinations or other psychotic symptoms.
- There is some evidence that delusional disorder may occur more often in individuals with ID [5, 6]. It is interesting to consider what factors may make this disorder more common in individuals with ID.
- There are several types of delusions that can be present.
  - Erotomanic—the individual believes that another person is in love with them when that person is not.
    - This can become confusing as it can be considered developmentally appropriate to have romantic or sexual feelings toward someone that the patient does not know, e.g., a movie star or a famous musician.

A helpful delineation for people with ID—as it is in people without—is that while it can be normal to have a crush on a famous person, the individual is able to recognize that the other person does not return those feelings.

- Individuals with ID can use magical thinking and fantasy as defenses, which mean that they can report being married to a famous person. If this is a helpful idea that increases coping, then it is likely not delusional disorder; however if this belief impacts social, emotional, or occupational functioning, it could be considered a disorder.

- Persecutory—the individual believes that others are out to harm them
- Grandiose—the individual believes that they are a very important or famous person.
  - While someone with delusional disorder does not need to have impaired functioning beyond the impact of the delusion, the individual might still encounter consequences [3].
  - An example is an individual who believes that he is Batman and declines work to be prepared to see the Bat Signal from the Commissioner.

Diagnosing Psychotic Disorders

Special care needs to be made to distinguish self-talk, traumatic re-experiencing, fantasy, and psychotic symptoms as well as ruling out any possible underlying medical or other psychiatric cause

- Self-talk is typically present at baseline and tends to increase during times of stress. Common topics can include conversations the individual has had over the course of the day, thinking out loud or repeating certain phrases. Self-talk typically does not include the individual listening as though they can hear someone speaking out loud to them.

- Traumatic re-experiencing, or flashbacks, are episodes where an individual feels as though they are re-experiencing a previous traumatic event.
  - A trauma history that includes the following information increases the clinician's ability to differentiate trauma symptoms like re-experiencing/flashbacks from psychotic symptoms such as hallucinations.
    - Known triggers—sights, smells, situations
    - Available details of trauma—people involved, location, surroundings
    - A timeline of the person's psychological and social history
- Fantasy is a coping style that is present in most individuals including persons with ID. This is not a psychotic symptom but rather an approach to the world that includes the magical thinking commonly associated with childhood where people have magical powers and abilities.
  - Clues in distinguishing this from psychotic symptoms are
    - Chronicity—these ideas are usually life-long.
    - Lack of impact on daily functioning—these characteristics tend to be coping skills that help a person make it through the day rather than impairments that impact quality of life and functional capacity.
- Because people with ID may have communication barriers, it is of utmost importance to rule out an underlying delirium, which is very often mistaken for psychosis. Delirium is an altered mental status due to an underlying medical condition like a urinary tract infection or pneumonia. The main differences include:
  - Delirium is typically of sudden onset while psychotic disorders, specifically schizophrenia, have a prodromal phase that can last months to years.
  - Delirium will wax and wane while psychotic symptoms remain fairly consistent.
  - Delirium typically involves predominantly visual hallucinations while psychotic disorders typically exhibit auditory hallucinations.
  - Sensorium is typically clouded in delirium.

- Obsessive compulsive disorder can present with unusual and difficult-to-understand symptoms such as ordering, tapping, or avoidance. Careful observation with context and situation can be useful in discerning obsessive compulsive disorder from psychotic disorders.

Treatment of Psychotic Disorder

After accurate diagnosis, including exclusion of medical etiologies of psychotic symptoms, an antipsychotic medication should be started at low dose and with slow increases until significant abatement of symptoms. First-line treatment includes second-generation antipsychotics or another antipsychotic that has previously been known to be effective and tolerated. Supportive psychotherapy including psycho-education is helpful for patients, families, and caregivers to manage symptoms that medications do not. Patients should be monitored for response and for side effects.

- Metabolic monitoring is necessary during use of antipsychotic medications as they impact carbohydrate metabolism as well as hunger and satiety. Measures needed are
  - Weight
  - Lipids including total cholesterol, HDL, triglycerides, and LDL
  - Blood glucose monitoring
- Tardive dyskinesia is a movement disorder than occurs in the general population but is thought to occur more frequently in those with ID as well as individuals who take antipsychotic medications. Monitoring is done with an Abnormal Involuntary Movement Scale (AIMS) every 3–6 months. The disorder is treated by lowering or stopping the antipsychotic, switching antipsychotics, or starting clozapine.
- Acute dystonia is the involuntary and painful tightening of one muscle or one group of muscles that occurs most commonly after initiation of antipsychotic medications. It can

be treated by using anticholinergics like benztropine or diphenhydramine.

- Parkinsonism is described as having masked facies (reduced facial expression), shuffling gait, and pill-rolling tremor. It can be ameliorated by reducing the dose of antipsychotics.
- Neuroleptic malignant syndrome is a potentially deadly side effect of antipsychotic medications. It is characterized by elevated body temperature, altered mental status, rigid muscles, and autonomic instability. Treatment is admission to the Intensive Care Unit, fluid resuscitation, and dantrolene or bromocriptine.
- Akathisia is a feeling of internal restlessness in which an individual describes the inability to sit or stand still. Individuals with this side effect often pace in place or move around restlessly.
- Sedation is the most common side effects of treatment with antipsychotic medication and tends to abate with time.

See Chap. 11 for further details on antipsychotic medications.

Conclusion

Individuals with intellectual disability have psychotic disorder symptoms that are close to those individuals without intellectual disability. If care is taken to make an appropriate diagnosis, treatment with antipsychotic medications should prove helpful.

Clinical Pearls
- Criteria for diagnosis remains largely unchanged for those with disabilities as those without.
- Coping styles like fantasy and self-talk should be considered before diagnosis.

- A diagnosis of psychotic disorder should include a change from baseline, which requires good collateral information from family and/or caregivers.
- Treatment for those with disabilities is similar to those without disabilities—the lowest effect dose of antipsychotic medication.
- Expressive language impairment can impair the reporting of side effects, so care should be taken to provide psychoeducation and monitoring.
- Other diagnoses like anxiety, post-traumatic stress disorder, obsessive compulsive disorder, and autism can present in similar manners and should be ruled out.

Case Vignette

Mr. A is a 25-year-old Caucasian man brought in by his mother and caregivers. He has diagnoses of mild intellectual disability and gastro-esophageal reflux disease. They report that over the last 6 months, he has started mentioning his movements are being monitored by "them." His mother reports that she is not aware of any monitoring but does report that he has been more withdrawn. He has been more reluctant to go to his day habilitation program and has not appeared to be as interested in his usual activities. She says that he has not seemed sad or "down," and she reports that he has not had any unusual events or big changes in his life. His caregiver reports that Mr. A started talking to himself and reports that Mr. A had never done this before. He reports overhearing Mr. A arguing and yelling, "No, leave me alone. Stop watching me." Mr. A reports that he knows people are watching and following him. When his mother and caregiver attempt to comfort him by telling him that he is not being followed, he became upset arguing, "I know they're following me!" A medical evaluation including MRI of his brain, metabolic panel, urinalysis and urine drug screen, complete blood count, and autoimmune panel were all negative. He was started on a low-dose, second-generation antipsychotic and responded well.

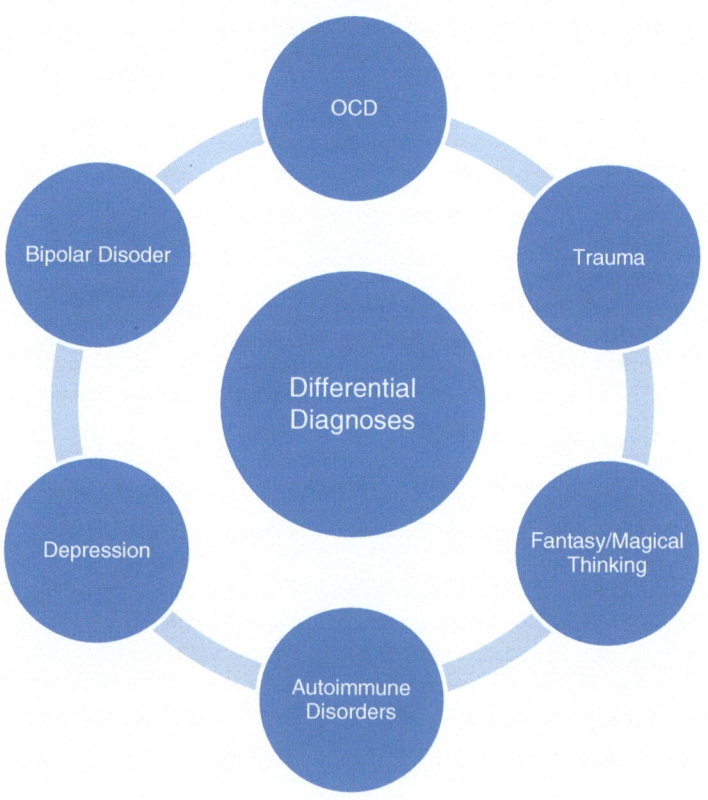

References

1. Deb S, Thomas M, Bright C. Mental disorder in adults with intellectual disability. 1: prevalence of functional psychiatric illness among a community-based population aged between 16 and 64 years. J Intellect Disabil Res. 2001;45(6):495–505.
2. Morgan VA, et al. Intellectual disability co-occurring with schizophrenia and other psychiatric illness: population-based study. Br J Psychiatry. 2008;193(5):364–72.
3. American Psychiatric Association. Diagnostic and statistical manual of mental disorders (DSM-5®). Washington, DC: American Psychiatric Pub; 2013.
4. Fletcher RJ, Barnhill J, Cooper SA. DM-ID-2: diagnostic manual-intellectual disability: a textbook of diagnosis of mental disorders in persons with intellectual disability. Kingston: National Assn for the Dually Diagnosed Press; 2016.
5. Williams H, et al. Use of the atypical antipsychotics olanzapine and risperidone in adults with intellectual disability. J Intellect Disabil Res. 2000;44(2):164–9.
6. Kishore MT, et al. Psychiatric diagnosis in persons with intellectual disability in India. J Intellect Disabil Res. 2004;48(1):19–24.

Chapter 10
Aggression

Kari Harper

Introduction

Aggression in its various forms (verbal, physical, property destruction, and autoaggression or self-injurious behavior) is the most frequent cause for mental health appointments and assessments in patients with intellectual disabilities (ID). Behavior changes and mental illness occur more frequently in individuals with ID, with nearly 1/3 exhibiting aggression or self-injurious behavior (SIB), and behavior changes are reported in 50–60%. Table 10.1 shows diagnostic criteria for problem behavior. Most aggressive events directed toward care staff are precipitated by denial of requests and often consist of verbal aggression alone. Nonetheless, careful evaluation and consideration of treatment of aggression is important. Impairment in communication may contribute to aggressive behavior in individuals with ID, and it is important

K. Harper (✉)
Wright State Psychiatry, Boonshoft School of Medicine, Wright State University, Dayton, OH, USA
e-mail: Kari.harper@wright.edu

© Springer Nature Switzerland AG 2019
J. P. Gentile et al. (eds.), *Guide to Intellectual Disabilities*,
https://doi.org/10.1007/978-3-030-04456-5_10

TABLE 10.1 Diagnostic criteria for problem behavior and self-injurious behavior (*Diagnostic Criteria for Psychiatric Disorders for Use with Adults with Learning Disabilities/Mental Retardation* [5])

General diagnostic criteria for problem behavior

    A. The problem behavior is of significant frequency, severity, or chronicity as to require clinical assessment and special interventions/support

    B. The problem behavior must not be a direct consequence of other psychiatric disorders, drugs, or physical disorders

    C. One of the following must be present:

1. The problem behavior results in a significant negative impact on the person's quality of life or quality of life of others. This may be owing to restriction of his or her lifestyle, social opportunities, independence, community integration, service access or choices, or adaptive functioning

2. The problem behavior presents significant risks to the health and/or safety of the person

    D. The problem behavior is pervasive. It is across a range of personal and social situations, although it may be more severe in certain identified settings

Self-injurious behavior

    A. The general diagnostic criteria for problem behavior are met

    B. Self-injury sufficient to cause tissue damage, such as bruising, scarring, tissue loss, and dysfunction, must have occurred during most weeks of the preceding 6-month period, e.g., ranging from skin-picking/scratching, hair-pulling, face slapping, to biting hands, lips, and other body parts, rectal/genital poking, eye-poking, and head banging

    C. The self-injurious behavior is not a deliberate suicide attempt

to consider possible causes for the aggression, including the need to communicate medical symptoms. Table 10.2 is a list of psychiatric and medical conditions associated with aggression [5].

TABLE 10.2 Summary of psychiatric and medical conditions associated with aggression [5]

Medical conditions
  Traumatic brain injury
  Intracranial pathology (trauma, infections, neoplasms, malformations)
  Cerebrovascular accidents
  Degenerative diseases
  Delirium
  Metabolic conditions (thyroid storm, Cushing syndrome, hormonal dysregulation, etc.)
  Systemic infections/local infections (i.e., otitis media, urinary tract infections, etc.)
  Environmental toxins
  Aberrant effects of medications
  Seizures, especially partial complex
  Sleep apnea
  Constipation
  Food and medication allergies
  Fractures
  Pain (acute and chronic, multiple etiologies)
Psychiatric conditions/symptoms
  Substance abuse disorders
  Psychotic disorders (especially paranoia)
  Affective disorders (especially mania, depression associated with irritability)
  Personality disorders (especially antisocial, borderline)
  Conduct disorder
  Oppositional defiant disorder
  Delirium, dementia
  Intellectual disability

Risk Factors

Many risk factors for aggression are common to both the general population and those with ID.

Static risk factors	Dynamic risk factors
Past violence	Persecutory delusions
Male gender	Command hallucinations
Younger adult age	Noncompliance
Cognitive deficits	Impulsivity
Brain injury	Low global assessment of functioning
Dissociative states	Homicidality
Military service	Depression
Weapons training	Hopelessness
Major mental illness	Suicidality
	Access to weapons

Some risk factors are unique to individuals with ID. SIB is related to more severe or profound ID, poorer communication skills, and autism. Sensory impairments and inability to express needs have been related to aggression and SIB. Aggression in children with ID is associated with co-occurring sleep problems, more severe ID, polypharmacy, seizure disorders, and cerebral palsy. Aggression toward others is more likely to be exhibited by persons with less severe cognitive deficits with greater verbal communication skills, while SIB is more common in individuals with severe ID, who may have decreased mobility, reduced self-help skills, more severe hearing impairment, increased stereotypic movements, and less well-developed communication skills [5].

Comorbid psychiatric and neurological disorders also confer additional risk for aggression and SIB. Psychiatric disorders associated with aggression in people with ID include impulse control disorders, stereotyped/habit disorders, anxiety disorders, mood disorders, psychotic symptoms/paranoia, and antisocial behaviors. SIB in particular can be a serious concern in patients with psychotic symptoms and paranoia. The prefrontal or frontal lobes, which play roles in executive functioning, logic and reasoning, and the temporal lobe, which plays a role in fear and response to danger, could affect aggression. Individuals with ID are more likely to have comorbid neurological disorders or dysfunctions, which affect these brain regions [5].

Times of transition are notoriously difficult for those with ID, and they experience many of them. Transitions may be related to educational or occupational settings, changes in family structure and dynamics, residential placements, and staff turnover. Individuals with ID may experience and re-experience grief and loss, and their families experience difficult transitions, grief, and loss as well. Furthermore, individuals may find that aggression is a powerful means of getting attention and communicating, and if it is more effective than other means of communication, treatment for aggression may not be effective [5].

Assessment: The Biopsychosocial Model

The biopsychosocial model is useful when attempting to determine the etiology of behavior change in a person with ID. It is important to gather information from the patient, family, caregivers, clinical records, and collaborating agencies. The assessment can evolve over time and incorporates supporting, predisposing, perpetuating, and protective factors related to the disorder. In the assessment of behavior change in an individual with ID, it is important to provide an environment most likely to de-escalate the situation. Use a calm, soothing tone, express concern, offer food or drink, allow trusted persons to be present when able, remove potentially dangerous objects, and distract with positive activities. Avoid overcrowding patients, exposing patients to loud noises, addressing only the caregiver, concealing hands in pockets, using intimidating direct eye contact or a confrontational stance, and unnecessarily invading personal space. It is important to talk both directly to the patient and to obtain collateral information from others present – this is often called "managing the triangle." Care in the approach to the situation can help the provider obtain accurate and complete information for the assessment [5].

Biological Component

The biological aspects of the assessment will include information such as:

- Demographics
- Medical history
- Genetic predispositions
- Family history
- Past and present medications
- Substance use

Especially important is a medication timeline and a medication history that includes medications the patient was taking at a time when he or she was doing well. The timeline is important, as patients with ID are more susceptible to medication side effects. It is also important to remember that aggression may be a way for a patient to communicate about a current medical illness, so documentation by caretaking staff of physical complaints, intake and output, sleep, appetite, energy level, toilet habits, and mood can be helpful to determine an underlying biological cause of the aggressive behavior. Table 10.3 lists possible biological interpretations of behavior change. Table 10.4 lists important laboratory values to be obtained when evaluating behavior change [5].

Psychological Component

Family history of violence, whether potentially genetically influenced or a learned behavior, is a predisposing factor, as patients who experience violence regularly at a young age are more likely to be aggressive. Psychological data obtained should also include:

- Abuse and trauma history
- Information about developmental years

TABLE 10.3 Common presentation of behavior problems and their possible meaning [5]

Fist jammed in mouth: consider gastroesophageal reflux disease, eruption of teeth, asthma, rumination, nausea, anxiety, painful hands, and gout

Biting side of hand: consider sinus problems, Eustachian tubes/ other ear problems, eruption of third molars, dental problems, pain or paresthesia of the hands

Biting object with front teeth: sinus problems [also the most common reason for thumb sucking and bruxism], Eustachian tube or ear problems, finger pain or paresthesia, and gout

Intense rocking: visceral pain, headache, depression, anxiety, or medication side effects

Refuses to sit evenly, or at all: hip pain, genital or rectal discomfort, clue to ongoing or past abuse

Unpleasurable masturbation: prostatitis, urinary tract or genital infection, rectal injury or infection, parasitic infection, syphilis or other "old" conditions, repetition phenomenon [past abuse], or never learned pleasurable masturbation

Waving head side to side: attempt to supplement visual field, vertigo, or hypervigilance

Walking on toes: arthritis in the hips, ankles, or knees, sensory integration issues or tight heel cords

Won't sit: akathisia, anxiety, depression, back pain or other pain, sleep deprivation

Whipping head forward: atlantoaxial subluxation [found in 14% of individuals with Down syndrome and others with joint laxity], dental problems, or headaches

Sudden sitting down or "sit down strikes": cardiac problems, syncope, orthostasis, medication side effects, vertigo, otitis, atlantoaxial subluxation, seizures, or panic

Waving fingers in front of eyes: migraine, corneal scarring, cataracts, seizures, glaucoma, or medication side effects, i.e., diplopia

Head banging: depression, headache, dental problems, seizures, otitis, mastoiditis, sinusitis, tinea capitis

TABLE 10.4 Laboratory evaluation of the patient with aggression [5]

Complete blood count

Electrolytes

Liver function

Renal function

Calcium level

Creatinine phosphokinase

Toxicology screen

Blood glucose level

CT or MRI (brain)

Optional tests: Any pertinent medication levels, ammonia level, antinuclear antibody, rheumatoid factor, sedimentation rate, thyroid function, chest radiograph, lipoprotein levels, B12 level, VDRL, arterial blood gases, additional medical or neurologic assessment (EEG, etc.) if indicated

- Institutionalizations
- Losses and history of change in caregiving staff
- Changes to environment
- Other significant changes that take place without warning
- Past counseling relationships
- Patient's coping skills

Patient's history of loss, turnover of caregivers, and changes in the environment may contribute to feelings of abandonment [5].

Social Component

Social outlets are important for people with ID, and it is imperative they feel safe in their environments [5]. Data should be gathered about:

- Residential placements
- Social activities
- Occupational/educational environments
- Hobbies and interests
- Spirituality

- Spending money
- Exercise and physical activity
- Feeling of safety

Treatment of Aggressive Behaviors

It is important to treat or attend to the underlying condition, whether that is a medical illness, a social situation, grief/loss, a psychiatric disorder, or other conditions identified by the biopsychosocial assessment. Targeted treatments yield better results [5].

Non-pharmacological Treatment

Since individuals with ID often have problems with executive functioning, it may be difficult for them to utilize cognitive components of various anger treatments, though if the core problem is maladaptive thoughts, a cognitive approach may be helpful. Non-cognitive components of various treatments – relaxation, self-monitoring, and skills training through role-play – may be most helpful. Various modalities of therapy have been instituted to treat aggression including behavioral, social skills training, cognitive, and group therapy [5]. CBT was shown to be effective in reducing aggression and physical assault in a population with mild or borderline ID in a forensic hospital setting [15]. In any case, it is important to manage both the feelings caregivers may have toward the patient and the provider's own countertransference. Caregivers may have fear or anger, and the provider could overestimate or underestimate risk, leading to over-involvement or becoming neglectful of the patient [5].

Pharmacological Treatment

Pharmacological treatments, particularly antipsychotic treatments, have been used inappropriately in the past for tranquilizing effects alone. It is important to remember that self-report of side effects could be compromised by limited communication abilities. It is estimated that 20% of individuals with ID experience adverse side effects and that some side effects, such as neuroleptic malignant syndrome, may manifest more severely [5]. Scheifes et al. [12] found that 84.4% of individuals with ID taking psychotropic medications experienced at least one adverse event, and almost half experienced three or more adverse events, with increased risk associated with polypharmacy. There may be metabolic, pharmacodynamic, and pharmacokinetic differences in individuals with ID as well as differences in drug reactions due to damage to the central nervous system (CNS). Treatment should be based on the most specific psychiatric diagnosis possible; however, medication treatment for individuals with ID often occurs without any documented psychiatric diagnosis other than ID and includes longer trials and polypharmacy. When pharmacological treatment is warranted, especially in children, starting doses of medication should be lower, and doses should be increased at slower rates. Furthermore, it is important to re-evaluate use of medications at regular intervals. It is also important to remember that some antipsychotics and antidepressants lower the seizure threshold, which is a common comorbidity in this population [5].

Antipsychotics: Adults

Antipsychotics are the most commonly used pharmacological treatment for aggression and behavior change in individuals with ID, ranging from 20% to 50%. In most studies, frequency and severity of aggression are decreased with use of antipsychotics. They are especially helpful when treating aggression associated with psychosis. It has been found that second-generation antipsychotics are as effective as first-generation antipsychotics in treating aggression but that weight gain and metabolic problems should be carefully monitored. Risperidone and olanzapine have been suggested as first-line agents, while quetiapine was suggested as a second-line agent [5]. A small study of aripiprazole in patients with fragile X syndrome showed a reduction in irritable behavior [4]. Evidence on use of aripiprazole shows benefits for treating aggression, including reduced aggression in populations with ID, developmental disability, and autism spectrum disorder and reduced rates of side effects compared to other antipsychotics [3]. Clozapine has been found to be helpful in reducing self-injury and in reducing aggression in patients for whom other pharmacological interventions have not been efficacious [5]. Benefits of use of antipsychotics also include reduction in use of restraint and seclusion [5]. Haloperidol has been repeatedly shown to be safe in treatment of acute violent behavior in individuals with ID, even if medical history is unknown [5]. Several studies have shown that antipsychotics can be successfully reduced and discontinued without return of aggressive behavior in 40–70% of the ID population [2, 8].

Antipsychotics: Children and Adolescents

Aripiprazole, asenapine, lurasidone, olanzapine, paliperidone, quetiapine and risperidone are approved for schizophrenia, bipolar mania, and/or bipolar depression in children and adolescents [14, 17]. Only aripiprazole and risperidone have been shown to have established efficacy and have FDA approval for treatment of irritability associated with ASD in children and adolescents [11]. Olanzapine may be useful in patients who do not find benefit with aripiprazole or risperidone, but weight gain is considerable [11]. Risperidone has been shown to have efficacy for treating hyperactivity, irritability, impulsivity, aggression against self and others and stereotypic behavior and that olanzapine had efficacy for treating hyperactivity and irritability [5]. Treatment with olanzapine, however, was associated with higher rates of side effects and dropout from the study [5]. Lurasidone has not been shown to be efficacious in treating aggression associated with autistic disorder in children and adolescents [7, 11]. Limited research has shown minimal efficacy and poor tolerability of quetiapine in treatment of children with pervasive developmental disability [11]. Paliperidone has also shown promise, and more studies are needed [11]. Ziprasidone has shown promise in some studies in treating irritability in the ID population; however, EKG monitoring is recommended, and there is concern for destabilization of underlying bipolar disorder [11]. Studies are needed to examine the efficacy of asenapine [11]. Clozapine has not been approved for the indication of disruptive behavior in children, and there is insufficient evidence for its efficacy [11]. Literature on the use of clozapine for treatment in patients less than 18 years of age is scarce [5].

Mood Stabilizers/Anticonvulsants: Adults

As seizure disorders are prevalent in the ID population, anticonvulsants/mood stabilizers are the second most common psychotropic medication class prescribed. Expert consensus guidelines list anticonvulsants/mood stabilizers as preferred medications for treatment of aggression and SIB. Sodium valproate was overwhelmingly the first choice. Approximately 70% of adults with ID and behavior changes showed improvement with sodium valproate. It is primarily used in conjunction with other agents at serum levels comparable to those used to treat seizures. Carbamazepine was the second choice of most expert consensus guidelines. There is some evidence for improvement of aggression for patients on topiramate, but overall evidence for use of topiramate in problem behaviors is lacking. Lithium has been shown to be effective for reducing aggression and irritability when used as an adjunct to other agents, especially in patients with bipolar disorder or older adults with psychosis. However, severe side effects have been reported, so treatment should be monitored carefully. Blood levels comparable to those needed to treat bipolar disorder were effective [5].

Mood Stabilizers/Anticonvulsants: Children and Adolescents

Sodium valproate is also the mood stabilizer of choice for treatment of aggression and SIB in children. Carbamazepine was shown to decrease agitation in children with brain injury. Lithium is not recommended for use in children under the age of 12 for any indication due to the increased risk of severe side effects [5].

Antidepressants: Adults

Individuals with low 5-hydroxyindoleacetic acid, a metabolite of serotonin, are more likely to exhibit aggression. Selective serotonin reuptake inhibitors (SSRIs) have established efficacy for decreasing aggression in general patients with various psychiatric diagnoses. Decreased aggression, SIB, destruction/disruption, and depression/dysphoria with the use of SSRIs and clomipramine have been reported. In people with ID, SSRIs have been found to decrease depression-related symptoms related to aggression, particularly with respect to SIB. An even higher percentage of patients with anxiety spectrum disorders treated with SSRIs showed significant improvement [5].

Antidepressants: Children

Though there are no specific guidelines for use of antidepressants to treat aggression in children and adolescents, there are antidepressants approved for treatment of depressive, anxiety, and obsessive-compulsive disorders in children including duloxetine, escitalopram, fluoxetine, fluvoxamine, and sertraline [16]. There is a black box warning for increased suicidal ideation with use of antidepressants in children and adolescents. Fluoxetine may have a positive effect on SIB, impulsivity, and depressive symptoms in children in ID. Use of antidepressants is associated with reduced stereotypic behaviors as well as improved communicative behaviors. There may be an increased risk of manic-like activation with the use of fluoxetine in some children with autistic disorder, so caution should be taken [5].

Other Medications and Biological Interventions

Research on opioid antagonists for treatment of impulsivity and aggression in adults reveals mixed results. Most adults experienced some short-term benefits, particularly with respect to SIB. It is theorized that SIB causes release of endogenous opioids that simultaneously stimulate the reward system in the CNS and calm the physical pain caused by the SIB, creating a cycle of behavior. Short-term, acute benefit of treatment with opioid antagonists for treatment of hyperactive, impulsive, stereotypic, and aggressive behavior has also been shown in children [5].

Benzodiazepines, which increase GABA, have anxiolytic and antiepileptic properties and may be used for a variety of conditions in the ID population, but low doses of shorter acting agents are recommended. The rate of side effects from benzodiazepines in this population is frequent and may include disinhibition, agitation, aggression, anger, depression, euphoria, and ataxia [5].

Beta-blockers, especially propranolol, have been used as an adjunct medication to help control violence, particularly in patients with traumatic brain injury. Beta-blockers decrease availability of norepinephrine, which may decrease aggression [5].

ADHD is more common in individuals with ID than in the general population, but patients with ID respond less well to psychostimulants than do the general population, though response rates were still found to be 45–65%. The strongest predictor of efficacy of a stimulant for aggression and disruptive behavior was IQ above 50. Individuals with ID experience more side effects related to stimulant use [5]. Atomoxetine, clonidine, and guanfacine, other medications often used to treat ADHD, have been shown to be efficacious in reducing irritability in the ID population with comorbid ADHD as well, though they are generally not as efficacious in treating ADHD as are stimulants [10]. Capone et al. [1] showed guanfacine was effective for reducing irritability and target behaviors associated with ADHD in children with Down syndrome and comorbid ADHD. Guanfacine was generally well tolerated. Clonidine was shown to improve sleep and decrease behavioral symptoms including aggression in children with ASD [9].

A case report has shown that acetylcysteine may be helpful as an adjunct treatment in reducing aggression and reducing the dose or frequency of other medications used to treat aggression [13].

Though an association between androgens and aggression has been well established, hormonal treatments are not recommended for use to decrease aggression due to lack of controlled studies and risk of serious side effects [5].

There are case studies showing increased mood stabilization, reduction in SIB and decreased behavioral disturbance in those with ID receiving ECT, but caution must be given with the increased prevalence of seizure disorders, lower rate of subjective side effect reporting, and complicated informed consent process [5]. A case report has also been described showing benefit of deep brain stimulation [6].

Summary of Treatment and Clinical Pearls

- De-escalate the situation using a calm environment. "Manage the triangle" between patient and caregivers.
- Attend to and treat underlying conditions.
- Relaxation techniques may be an effective intervention that can be taught and utilized to reduce aggressive behaviors.
- Individuals with ID are more susceptible to side effects of medications and adverse events and less able to communicate side effects than the general population.
- Start with low doses of medications and increase slowly, particularly in children.

- Re-evaluate use of medications regularly, and decrease dose or frequency and discontinue use as able.
- Use of psychotropic medications is most effective when targeting a specific psychiatric diagnosis.
- Antipsychotics are the most common psychotropic medications used for aggression and behavior change in individuals with ID. Second-generation antipsychotics are as effective as first-generation antipsychotics with fewer side effects, but metabolic parameters should be monitored.
- Aripiprazole and risperidone have been FDA approved to treat irritability associated with ASD in children and adolescents.
- Haloperidol is safe and effective in emergency situations.
- Both antipsychotics and antidepressants may lower the seizure threshold.
- Mood stabilizers/anticonvulsants, particularly sodium valproate, have been found to be effective in treating aggression.
- Lithium is shown to reduce aggression and irritability as an adjunct to other agent especially in adults with bipolar disorder or older adults with psychosis.
- Antidepressants may have particular efficacy in treating underlying anxiety disorders and reducing self-injury.
- Treating comorbid ADHD is important though not as successful as treating ADHD in the general population.
- Medications targeting the noradrenergic system, such as beta-blockers, guanfacine and clonidine, may be helpful in treating aggression, especially in an adjunctive capacity.
- Newer antipsychotics as well as other treatments such as acetylcysteine, ECT, and DBS need further study.
- Hormonal treatments have not been shown to be effective, and side effects can be severe.

Clinical Vignette [5]
Mary Jane was a 23-year-old female with history of severe intellectual disability and bipolar disorder. She

presented for mental health assessment for mood cycling, episodic agitation, and head banging. The patient had transitioned from an educational setting to her occupational setting about 3 months earlier; the staff reported that the transition had gone smoothly. She had begun banging her head on walls and tables in both her work and home environments about 2 weeks prior to the mental health assessment. She reportedly had decreased appetite and had lost approximately 2 pounds in the last 2 weeks. She also had episodes of crying which appeared to be random and not precipitated by any external factor. The patient was not aggressive toward others and did not destroy property. She seemed inconsolable during the head banging episodes, and staff was at a loss of how to assist. Her medication regimen included valproate (Depakote), quetiapine (Seroquel), and buspirone (Buspar). Her bipolar disorder had been stable on this medication regimen for approximately 10 months. Her medical history was significant for diagnosis of gastroesophageal reflux disease and allergic rhinitis; however, she was not on any prescription medication for either condition. The patient was nonverbal, and so all information was gathered by collateral data sources including direct care staff at both work and home settings. The patient had no family involvement. It was recommended that the patient receive a thorough physical exam by her primary care physician and to address the question of potential treatment for the reflux disease and allergic rhinitis. A dental examination to rule out oral cavity problems was also recommended since the head and neck areas were directly involved. Because the patient presented with head banging other conditions significant to be ruled out included depression, headache syndromes, dental problems, seizure disorders, otitis/sinusitis, and other upper respiratory problems. At the dental appointment, Mary Jane received oral x-rays that revealed the impending eruption of her third molars. The surgical procedure was scheduled and conducted within 1 week. The head banging resolved after recovery from the surgical procedure.

References

1. Capone GT, Brecher L, Bay M. Guanfacine use in children with down syndrome and comorbid attention-deficit hyperactivity disorder (ADHD) with disruptive behaviors. J Child Neurol. 2016;31(8):957–64. https://doi.org/10.1177/0883073816634854.
2. de Kuijper G, Evenhuis H, Minderaa RB, Hoekstra PJ. Effects of controlled discontinuation of long-term used antipsychotics for behavioural symptoms in individuals with intellectual disability. J Intellect Disabil Res. 2014;58(1):71–83. https://doi.org/10.1111/j.1365-2788.2012.01631.x.
3. Deb S, Farmah BK, Arshad E, Deb T, Roy M, Unwin GL. The effectiveness of aripiprazole in the management of problem behaviour in people with intellectual disabilities, developmental disabilities and/or autistic spectrum disorder--a systematic review. Res Develop Disabil. 2014;35(3):711–25. https://doi.org/10.1016/j.ridd.2013.12.004.
4. Erickson CA, Stigler KA, Wink LK, Mullett JE, Kohn A, Posey DJ, McDougle CJ. A prospective open-label study of aripiprazole in fragile X syndrome. Psychopharmacology. 2011;216(1):85–90. https://doi.org/10.1007/s00213-011-2194-7.
5. Gentile JP, Gillig PM, editors. Psychiatry of intellectual disability: a practical manual. Hoboken: John Wiley & Sons; 2012.
6. Harat M, Rudas M, Zielinski P, Birska J, Sokal P. Deep brain stimulation in pathological aggression. Stereotact Funct Neurosurg. 2015;93(5):310–5. https://doi.org/10.1159/000431373.
7. Loebel A, Brams M, Goldman RS, Silva R, Hernandez D, Deng L, Mankoski R, Findling RL. Lurasidone for the treatment of irritability associated with autistic disorder. J Autism Dev Disord. 2016;46(4):1153–63. https://doi.org/10.1007/s10803-015-2628-x.

8. McNamara R, Randell E, Gillespie D, Wood F, Felce D, Romeo R, Angel L, Espinasse A, Hood K, Davies A, Meek A, Addison K, Jones G, Deslandes P, Allen D, Knapp M, Thapar A, Kerr M. A pilot randomised controlled trial of community-led ANtipsychotic drug REduction for adults with learning disabilities. Health Technol Assess (Winchester, England). 2017;21(47):1–92. https://doi.org/10.3310/hta21470.

9. Ming X, Gordon E, Kang N, Wagner GC. Use of clonidine in children with autism spectrum disorders. Brain Dev. 2008;30(7):454–60. https://doi.org/10.1016/j.braindev.2007.12.007.

10. Patel BD, Barzman DH. Pharmacology and pharmacogenetics of pediatric ADHD with associated aggression: a review. Psychiatr Q. 2013;84(4):407–15. https://doi.org/10.1007/s11126-013-9253-7.

11. Politte LC, McDougle CJ. Atypical antipsychotics in the treatment of children and adolescents with pervasive developmental disorders. Psychopharmacology. 2014;231(6):1023–36. https://doi.org/10.1007/s00213-013-3068-y.

12. Scheifes A, Walraven S, Stolker JJ, Nijman HL, Egberts TC, Heerdink ER. Adverse events and the relation with quality of life in adults with intellectual disability and challenging behaviour using psychotropic drugs. Res Dev Disabil. 2016;49-50:13–21. https://doi.org/10.1016/j.ridd.2015.11.017.

13. Stutzman D, Dopheide J. Acetylcysteine for treatment of autism spectrum disorder symptoms. Am J Health-Syst Pharm. 2015;72(22):1956–9. https://doi.org/10.2146/ajhp150072.

14. Sunovion receives FSA approval of supplemental new drug application (SNDA) for use of latuda® (LURASIDONE HCI) in the treatment of bipolar depression in pediatric patients (10 to 17 years of age) (2018). Retrieved from http://news.sunovion.com/press-release/sunovion-receives-fda-approval-supplemental-new-drug-application-snda-use-latuda

15. Taylor JL, Novaco RW, Brown T. Reductions in aggression and violence following cognitive behavioural anger treatment for detained patients with intellectual disabilities. J Intellect Disabil Res. 2016;60(2):126–33. https://doi.org/10.1111/jir.12220.

16. U. S. Department of Health and Human Services, Centers for Medicare and Medicaid Services. (2015). Antidepressant medications: use in pediatric patients. Retrieved from https://www.cms.gov/Medicare-Medicaid-Coordination/Fraud-Prevention/

Medicaid-Integrity-Education/Pharmacy-Education-Materials/
Downloads/ad-pediatric-factsheet11-14.pdf
17. U.S. Department of Health and Human Services, Centers
for Medicare and Medicaid Services. (2013). Atypical antipsychotic medications: use in pediatric patients. Retrieved
from https://www.cms.gov/Medicare-Medicaid-Coordination/
Fraud-Prevention/Medicaid-Integrity-Education/Pharmacy-
Education-Materials/Downloads/atyp-antipsych-pediatric-fact-
sheet11-14.pdf

Chapter 11
Psychotropic Medications in Individuals with Intellectual Disability

David W. Dixon

General Guiding Principles

- Have a clear plan in place when starting psychotropic medications.
  - Establish a baseline of symptoms and behaviors that will be targeted before initiating therapy.
    - Document symptoms.
    - Consider rating scales for patients with better developed communication skills.
  - Discuss the expected effects from the medication.
    - Communicate a timeframe for onset of potential medication adverse effects (potentially quicker onset) and anticipated therapeutic benefits (potentially later onset) [1].

D. W. Dixon (✉)
San Antonio Military Medical Center, Houston, TX, USA
e-mail: david.dixon@wright.edu

© Springer Nature Switzerland AG 2019
J. P. Gentile et al. (eds.), *Guide to Intellectual Disabilities*,
https://doi.org/10.1007/978-3-030-04456-5_11

- Involve the patient, caregiver, and multidisciplinary team in discussions about expectations from medications.
  - Provide a plan for potential alternative strategies if desired effects are not fully realized or if symptoms fail to improve.
    - Trials of psychotropic medications in persons with ID may take a longer period of time [2].
  - Obtain baseline lab testing when initiating treatments, and update yearly as recommended for individual medications or classes. Consider increasing laboratory protocols for closer monitoring.
  - Consider dosing strategies that simplify regimens when possible and maximize secondary beneficial effects.
    - Opt for once-a-day dosing or extended release formulations when available.
    - Explore the patient's ability to take medications and adjust accordingly.
      - Difficulty with pill swallowing is common. Consider ordering liquid formulations, capsules, fast-melting tablets, or tablets that can be crushed when necessary.
    - Use more sedating medications at night to improve sleep.
      - Minimize the use of sedating medications during the day.
      - Anxiolytic effects can sometimes be achieved with much lower daytime dosing without causing significant sedation.
    - Utilize activating medications in the morning and avoid dosing too close to bedtime.
      - Consider effects on sleep, weight, appetite, and smoking status
    - Involve the multidisciplinary team when choosing dosing strategies [2].
      - A patient's symptoms may change throughout the course of the day and especially between changing environments, understanding which behaviors are present in different environments will assist with

optimization of medication timing. Dosing in mid-afternoon at the time of transition from structured environments to home may be very helpful.

- Initiate medications at low doses, titrate at a slower rate, and utilize maintenance or maximum doses at or below those used by the general population.
  - Medication adjustments should only be made when necessary (i.e., adverse effects, poor response), gradually, and with as few medications as possible.
  - Medications should be titrated to maximum beneficial effect, without exceeding maximum dosing recommendations, and evaluated for efficacy every 1–3 months, with the goal of lowering doses whenever possible to maintain therapeutic benefits while minimizing adverse effects and medication burden.
- Evaluation of beneficial and adverse effects should be performed at each visit.
  - Utilize baseline symptom data to evaluate changes to determine whether a medication adjustment is warranted (i.e., titrating medications to maximize improvements and tapering medications not having desired effects).
  - Monitor for any changes to patient's functional status (i.e., cognition, ability to participate in workshops, sedation, sleeping patterns, or appetite).
  - Patients with ID are more vulnerable to side effects than those in the general population.
  - Discuss behavioral changes that may represent side effects. Refer to Chap. 12 for more information.
- Utilize as few medications as possible to fully treat targeted symptoms.
  - Avoid polypharmacy.
  - Consider switching medications within the same class if therapeutic benefits are not demonstrated at modest doses.

  - Maximize therapeutic benefits from one medication before augmenting with another by judiciously titrating and evaluating benefits.
  - Using medications from multiple classes or multiple medications from a single class warrants justification by diagnosis or suboptimal response to single medications.
  - Openly discuss social concerns, substance use/abuse, medication adherence, sleeping patterns, nutritional status, physical activity, medical conditions, treatment expectations, and side effects.
- Reevaluate the plan throughout the course of treatment.
  - Utilize baseline symptom data and rating scales when re-assessing treatment strategies.
  - Discuss subjective and objective accounts of behaviors and symptoms from the past and present when discussing the efficacy of medications.
  - Reiterate the current plan and discuss any modifications that may arise from the "lessons learned" throughout the course of treatment.
  - Remain flexible with a willingness to work with the patient, caregiver, and multidisciplinary team to address concerns regarding medications, side effects, dosing strategies, behavioral interventions, and social interventions [1].

Psychotropic Medications

Antidepressants

- Selective serotonin reuptake inhibitors (SSRIs)—While the evidence is unclear for the use of SSRIs in the treatment of behavioral problems in patients with ID, SSRIs remain a safe and effective way to treat depressive, anxiety, obsessive-compulsive, and post-traumatic stress disorders.

All antidepressants currently hold a Food and Drug Administration (FDA) black box warning for the emergence of suicidal risk in children, adolescents, and young adults with major depressive or other psychiatric disorders which should be related to any patient under the age of 24 years and that patient's guardian.

- Fluoxetine, sertraline, citalopram, escitalopram, and paroxetine are commonly prescribed SSRIs.
  - Recommend low starting dose.
  - Typically prescribed once daily, preferably in the morning with food as GI effects and activation are common.
  - Pearls:
    - Sedation is rare; if present, change to evening dosing before discontinuation.
    - Often have liquid formulations available.
    - Citalopram—but not escitalopram—carries a warning for QT prolongation with higher doses.
    - Can often take 2–6 weeks for full effect.
    - Paroxetine has a shorter half-life, which can lead to discontinuation syndrome in the case of abrupt discontinuation.
  - Recommended labs/monitoring:
    - Standard baseline labs for ID population (CMP, CBC w/Diff, TSH, Beta hCG)
    - Baseline EKG
    - Monitor weight
- Serotonin and norepinephrine reuptake inhibitors (SNRIs):
  - Venlafaxine extended release, desvenlafaxine, and duloxetine are commonly prescribed SNRIs.
  - Recommend a low starting dose.
  - Pearls:
    - Can take 2–6 weeks to see full effect.
    - May be helpful with neuropathic pain.
    - Discontinuation syndrome can be uncomfortable.
    - May be of some benefit in attentional symptoms.

- Recommended labs and monitoring:
  - Baseline EKG
  - Monitor weight
  - Baseline and frequent blood pressure checks
- Atypical antidepressants:
  - Bupropion, extended release:
    - Pearls:
      - May be beneficial for assistance with smoking cessation.
      - May be beneficial as augmenting agent to SSRIs.
      - Contraindicated for use of immediate-release formulation with eating disorders.
      - Caution if seizure disorder exists.
      - Can be activating.
      - Less likely to cause sexual side effects than other antidepressants; in some cases it may improve this side effect.
  - Mirtazapine:
    - Pearls:
      - Weight gain is a very common side effect, so monitor diet/exercise when possible.
      - May be beneficial as augmenter to SSRI or SNRI-induced insomnia or anxiety.
      - Less likely to cause sexual side effects than other antidepressants.
      - All tablets are crushable.
  - Buspirone:
    - Buspirone is an anxiolytic that functions as a partial agonist at the Serotonin 1A receptor. It has demonstrated efficacy in persons with ID especially for anxiety symptoms and may be a good augmenting agent for antidepressants when dealing with comorbid anxiety and depression.
    - Pearls:
      - All tablets are scored and crushable.
      - Works best as augmenting agent for anxiety and depression [3–7].

Antipsychotics

- Atypical antipsychotics (second-generation antipsychotics; SGAs):
  - There are specific patient monitoring guidelines recommended for the use of all antipsychotics that should not be ignored prior to initiating treatment. In general, the use of antipsychotic medications should be reserved for patient suffering from psychotic and/or manic symptoms or under circumstances where benefits outweigh risks like acute agitation or severe self-injury. All antipsychotics can lower seizure threshold, carry the risk of neuroleptic malignant syndrome, painful dystonic reactions, metabolic syndrome, and other serious side effects [3–7].
  - Aripiprazole
    - FDA indicated to treat psychotic symptoms related to schizophrenia and manic symptoms related to bipolar disorders. It is also indicated to treat the irritability associated with autism spectrum in children. It can also be used to augment antidepressant effects in treating depression.
      - Available in depot formulation (requires oral dosing to establish tolerability, then overlapping oral medication for 14 days after initial injection)
      - Oral solution and orally disintegrating tablets are available.
    - Recommended Labs/Monitoring:
      - Standard baseline labs for antipsychotic use (CMP, CBC w/Diff, TSH, HgBA1c, Fasting Lipids, Beta hCG) should be performed at least annually; consider bi-annually in ID.
      - Annual EKG.
      - Monitor weight and abdominal circumference.
      - AIMS test at baseline, after adjustments, and every 6 months.

- Pearls:
  - Akathisia may develop during rapid titration or higher doses. Titrate slowly. This can mimic agitation, mania, and anger.
  - Avoid using for those at risk of developing hypotension.
  - May be less sedating than other SGAs.
- Risperidone
  - FDA indicated to treat psychotic symptoms related to schizophrenia and manic symptoms related to bipolar disorder. It is indicated to treat the irritability associated with autism in children.
  - Available in depot formulation, orally disintegrating tablets and liquid as well as pills
  - Recommended labs and monitoring
    - Standard baseline labs for antipsychotic use should be performed at least annually.
    - Annual EKG.
    - Monitor weight and abdominal circumference.
    - AIMS test at baseline, after adjustments, and every 6 months.
  - Pearls:
    - Dystonia may develop during rapid titration. Titrate slowly.
    - Avoid using for those at risk of developing hypotension.
    - Caution with renal/hepatic impairment.
    - Prolactin elevations are common; monitor and include an informed consent process.
- Quetiapine and olanzapine and other second-generation antipsychotics
  - Same testing as above is recommended
- Pearls
  - Can be sedating but should not be used to treat primary insomnia
  - May require twice daily dosing due to sedation
  - Caution for hypotension
  - Weight gain can be significant
- Typical antipsychotics, also known as first-generation antipsychotics

- While they are becoming less common in psychiatric practice due to the relative efficacy and safety of the SGA, patients with ID are still prescribed some of these medications.
- If one of these medications has been immensely helpful for a patient, a discussion of the risks and benefits of continuing treatment should cover newer alternatives but ultimately the decision about continuing pharmacotherapy should be a collaborative agreement among the patient, caregivers, and clinician [3–7].

Attention Deficit Hyperactivity Disorder (ADHD) Treatments

- Stimulants—Stimulants are commonly used to treat ADHD in children and adults. Approved age ranges vary depending on the medication and formulation. The goal of treatment is symptomatic relief of ADHD symptoms such as inattentiveness, hyperactivity, or poor concentration with treatment continued indefinitely while improvement is maintained.
  - Pearls for treatment:
    - Weight loss is common.
    - Effects may not be seen with initial dosing but can require careful titration to maximize benefit.
    - May cause anxiety, tremors, tachycardia, hypertension, and adverse cardiac symptoms.
    - Avoid use in those at risk of substance disorder.
    - Contraindicated in those with cardiac abnormalities.
    - No response or poor response may warrant switching to methylphenidate or a non-stimulant. Failing those, reconsider diagnosis or search for co-occurring disorder.
  - Recommended labs and monitoring:
    - Annual and baseline EKG; assess for cardiac disease history.
    - Monitor blood pressure regularly.
    - Standard baseline labs for ID patients (CMP, CBC w/ Diff, TSH, Beta hCG) should be performed at least annually.

- Non-stimulants—Can be used as monotherapy or as augmenting agents for stimulants when treating ADHD. The tolerability, efficacy, and mechanism of action vary greatly between the different agents and should help to guide prescribers when determining the most appropriate treatment for patients with ID and ADHD. The abuse potential of these medications, when compared to stimulants, may make them more favorable for those at risk for substance use disorders.
  - Guanfacine:
    - Guanfacine acts on the alpha-2A receptors in the prefrontal cortex, with higher selectivity than for the alpha-2B or alpha-2C receptors. Used to treat high blood pressure. Commonly used to treat concentration, motor hyperactivity, and impulsive behaviors seen in ADHD. Approved for use in children aged 6–17 years. Some efficacy to decrease tics with Tourette syndrome or other tic disorders.
      - Allow 3–4 weeks between changes.
    - Recommended labs/monitoring:
      - Standard baseline labs for ID patients (CMP, CBC w/Diff, TSH, Beta hCG) should be performed at least annually.
      - Annual EKG
      - Monitor blood pressure (hypotension common) and vitals regularly
    - Pearls:
      - Sedation is common.
      - Dose-related side effects with sinus bradycardia and hypotension can be especially concerning to patients and caregivers.
      - Use low dosing for renal impairment.
    - Use caution with hepatic impairment or cardiac abnormalities.
  - Atomoxetine:
    - Atomoxetine acts to block the reuptake of norepinephrine in the prefrontal cortex with some secondary increase in dopamine as well. It is used to treat symptoms related to ADHD in adults and children. It may also be used to treat depression.

- Pearls:
  - Sedation is common.
  - Do not use in persons with acute angle closure glaucoma.
  - Caution with hepatic impairment.
  - Do not use when cardiac abnormalities are present.
- Bupropion [see above] [3–7]

Hypnotic Sedatives

- Melatonin and ramelteon:
  - Allow at least 1 week between changes.
  - May cause respiratory depression in conjunction with other central nervous system depressants.
  - Little concern for contributing to or to developing a substance use disorder.
- Benzodiazepines:
  - Benzodiazepines may impact the patient's memory and cognitive sensorium.
  - They may cause suppression of the respiratory drive.
  - They can lead to physiologic dependence and tolerance. There may also be a paradoxical impact on patients with ID, resulting in disorientation and disinhibition, which may exacerbate problems with agitation and impulse control. In general, it is best to work toward reducing or eliminating the use of benzodiazepines in this population and reserve their use for very specific circumstances [3–7].

Mood Stabilizers/Anticonvulsants

- Lithium is the oldest of the known mood stabilizers and is used to treat mania, hypomania, bipolar depression, or as maintenance treatment.
  - Recommended labs and monitoring:
    - Standard baseline labs for ID patients (CMP, CBC w/ Diff, TSH, Beta hCG) performed at least annually

- Monitoring for diabetes insipidus
- Monitor blood pressure (hypotension common) and vitals regularly
- Regular monitoring of drug levels—trough levels:
  - Augmentation: 0.4–0.8 mmol/L
  - Monotherapy: 0.8–1.0 mmol/L
  - Toxicity is potentially fatal and should be treated with inpatient dialysis and monitoring
- Common side effects include sedation, cognitive slowing, tremor, weight gain, acne and increased urination.
- Valproic acid is a mood stabilizer and an antiepileptic.
  - Recommended labs and monitoring—see above:
    - Regular monitoring of drug levels—also trough levels:
      - Monotherapy: 70–100 mcg/mL
  - This medication is a known teratogen and women of child-bearing age should be counseled accordingly.
  - Care should be taken when using concurrently with lamotrigine.
  - Common side effects include sedation, tremor, cognitive slowing, and weight gain. It carries a warning for sudden hepatic failure.
- Carbamazepine is also a mood stabilizer and an antiepileptic.
  - Recommended labs and monitoring—see above:
    - Regular monitoring of drug levels:
      - Monotherapy: 7–12 mcg/mL
  - Common side effects include sedation and fatigue.
- Lamotrigine is also a mood stabilizer and an antiepileptic.
  - There is a precise, slow titration schedule as quick titrations have been connected with the development of the potentially fatal Stevens Johnson syndrome.
    - This medication does not require monitoring levels.
- Other antiepileptics such as oxcarbazepine, topiramate, gabapentin, and pregabalin are used as mood stabilizers. Each has also demonstrated various levels of efficacy in stabilization of mood with bipolar disorder in off-label use. If these medications are prescribed, they should be considered on a case-by-case basis [3–7].

Alphabetical Med List

Class	Subclass	Name	Generic?	Suggested starting dose for ID/DD	Effective range	Labs/studies	Serious S/E	Notes
ADHD	Nonstimulant	Guanfacine	Yes	1 mg bedtime	5–7 mg/day	EKG, standard + BP monitoring	Sinus bradycardia, hypotension	
ADHD	NRI	Atomoxetine	Yes	40 mg daily	40–100 mg/day	EKG, standard + BP monitoring	HTN, orthostatic hypotension, liver damage	
ADHD	Stimulant	Amphetamine (d,l)	Yes	5 mg daily	5–40 mg/day	EKG, standard + BP monitoring	Seizures, cardiac abnormalities	
ADHD	Stimulant	Lisdexamfetamine	No	30 mg daily	30–70 mg/day	EKG, standard + BP monitoring	Seizures, cardiac abnormalities	
ADHD	Stimulant	Methylphenidate v(d,l)	Yes	20 mg daily	20–60 mg/day	EKG, standard + BP monitoring	Seizures, cardiac abnormalities	
Alcohol dependence treatment	Mu opioid receptor antagonist	Naltrexone	Yes	25 mg daily	50 mg/day	Standard	Eosinophilic pneumonia, hepatocellular Injury (excessive doses)	
Alcohol dependence treatment		Acamprosate	Not in USA	333 mg tid	666 mg tid	Standard	Suicidal Ideation/ behavior	Decrease dose for renal impairment
Alcohol dependence treatment		Disulfiram	Yes	250 mg	250–500 mg/day	Standard + LFT monitoring	Hepatotoxicity, cardiac abnormalities	

(continued)

Class	Subclass	Name	Generic?	Suggested starting dose for ID/DD	Effective range	Labs/studies	Serious S/E	Notes
Anticholinergic		Benztropine	Yes	0.5 mg daily	1–4 mg/day	Standard	Angle closure glaucoma, cardiac arrhythmias, urinary retention	
Anticholinergic	Antiparkinson agent	Trihexyphenidyl	Yes	1 mg daily	1–15 mg/day divided	Standard	Angle closure glaucoma, cardiac arrhythmias, urinary retention	
Anticonvulsant	A2D Ligand	Gabapentin	Yes	Varies	Varies	Extensive	Aplastic anemia, agranulocytosis, SJS, SIADH	Psychiatrist/ neurologist oversight recommended
Anticonvulsant	A2D Ligand	Pregabalin	Yes	Varies	Varies	Extensive		Psychiatrist/ neurologist oversight recommended
Anticonvulsant	SGRI	Tiagabine	Yes	Varies	Varies	Extensive		Psychiatrist/ neurologist oversight recommended
Anticonvulsant	VSSC	Topiramate	Yes	Varies	Varies	Extensive		Psychiatrist/ neurologist oversight recommended

Class	Mechanism	Medication		Dose	Dose/day	Monitoring	Warnings	Oversight
Anticonvulsant	VSSC	Zonisamide	Yes	Varies	Varies	Extensive	Aplastic anemia, agranulocytosis, SJS, SIADH	Psychiatrist/neurologist oversight recommended
Anticonvulsant		Levetiracetam	Yes	Varies	Varies	Extensive		Psychiatrist/neurologist oversight recommended
Antidepressant	A2 antagonist	Mirtazapine	Yes	7.5 mg bedtime	45 mg/day	Standard + weight monitoring	Black box warning (SI), seizure	
Antidepressant	MAOI	Isocarboxazid	Not in USA	10 mg BID	40–60 mg/day	Standard + BP monitoring + weight monitoring	Hypertensive crisis, suicidal ideation, seizures, hepatotoxicity	MAOI diet required
Antidepressant	MAOI	Phenelzine	Yes	15 mg TID	45–75 mg/day	Standard + BP monitoring + weight monitoring		MAOI diet required
Antidepressant	MAOI	Selegiline	Yes	Varies	Varies	Standard + BP monitoring + weight monitoring		MAOI diet required
Antidepressant	Multimodal	Vortioxetine	No	5 mg	5–20 mg/day	Standard	Seizure, SI	

(continued)

Class	Subclass	Name	Generic?	Suggested starting dose for ID/DD	Effective range	Labs/studies	Serious S/E	Notes
Antidepressant	NDRI	Bupropion	Yes	(a) 375 mg BID for immediate-release (b) 100 mg BID for sustained-release (c) 150 mg daily for extended-release	(a) 225–450 mg in 3 divided doses for immediate-release (b) 200–450 mg in 2 divided doses for sustained-release (c) 150–450 mg once daily for extended-release	Standard + EKG	Black box warning (SI), seizure	
Antidepressant	SARI	Nefazodone	Yes	50 mg BID	300–600 mg/day divided	Standard	Black box warning (SI), seizure, hepatic failure, priapism	
Antidepressant	SARI	Trazodone	Yes	25 mg QHS	150–600 mg/day	Standard	Black box warning (SI), seizure, priapism	
Antidepressant	SNRI	Desvenlafaxine	No	50 mg	50–100 mg/day	Standard + BP monitoring	Black box warning (SI), seizure	
Antidepressant	SNRI	Duloxetine	Yes	20 mg BID	40–60 mg/day	Standard + BP monitoring	Black box warning (SI), seizure	

Antidepressant	SNRI	Levomilnacipran	No	20 mg	40–120 mg/day	Standard + BP/HR monitoring	Black box warning (SI), seizure
Antidepressant	SNRI	Milnacipran	No	12.5 mg	30–200 mg/day divided	Standard + BP monitoring	Black box warning (SI), seizure
Antidepressant	SNRI	Venlafaxine	Yes	(a) 25–50 mg BID for immediate-release (b) 37.5 mg daily for extended-release	(a) 75–225 mg in 2–3 divided doses for immediate-release (b) 75–225 mg daily for extended-release	Standard + BP monitoring	Black box warning (SI), seizure
Antidepressant	SPARI	Vilazodone	No	10 mg	40 mg/day	Standard	Black box warning (SI), seizure
Antidepressant	SSRI	Citalopram	Yes	10 mg	10–40 mg	Standard	Black box warning (SI), seizure
Antidepressant	SSRI	Escitalopram	Yes	5 mg	10–20 mg	Standard	Black box warning (SI), seizure
Antidepressant	SSRI	Fluoxetine	Yes	10 mg	20–80 mg	Standard	Black box warning (SI), seizure
Antidepressant	SSRI	Fluvoxamine	Yes	25 mg	50–300 mg/day	Standard	Black box warning (SI), seizure

(continued)

138 D. W. Dixon

Class	Subclass	Name	Generic?	Suggested starting dose for ID/DD	Effective range	Labs/studies	Serious S/E	Notes
Antidepressant	SSRI	Paroxetine	Yes	10 mg	20–50 mg/day	Standard	Black box warning (SI), seizure	
Antidepressant	SSRI	Sertraline	Yes	25 mg	50–200 mg/day	Standard	Black box warning (SI), seizure	
Antidepressant	TCA	Amitriptyline	Yes	25 mg QHS	Up to 300 mg/day in divided doses	EKG, standard + weight monitoring	Hyperthermia, seizure, cardiac anomalies, hepatic failure, increased IOP	Cardiac and hepatic concerns
Antidepressant	TCA	Clomipramine	Yes	25 mg	100–250 mg/day	EKG, standard + weight monitoring	Hyperthermia, seizure, cardiac anomalies, hepatic failure, increased IOP	
Antidepressant	TCA	Desipramine	Yes	25 mg	75–300 mg/day divided	EKG, standard + weight monitoring	Hyperthermia, seizure, cardiac anomalies, hepatic failure, increased IOP	
Antidepressant	TCA	Doxepin	Yes	25 mg	75–150 mg/day divided	EKG, standard + weight monitoring	Hyperthermia, seizure, cardiac anomalies, hepatic failure, increased IOP	

Antidepressant	TCA	Imipramine	Yes	25 mg QHS	50–150 mg/day	EKG, standard + weight monitoring	Hyperthermia, seizure, cardiac anomalies, hepatic failure, increased IOP
Antidepressant	TCA	Nortriptyline	Yes	10 mg QHS	75–150 mg/day daily or divided	EKG, standard + weight monitoring	Hyperthermia, seizure, cardiac anomalies, hepatic failure, increased IOP
Antihistamine	Anticholinergic	Diphenhydramine	Yes	25 mg	25–50 mg/day	Standard	Urinary retention, cardiac abnormalities, confusion/delirium
Antihypertensive	A1 adrenergic blocker	Prazosin	Yes	1 mg	1–16 mg/day divided	Standard	Syncope with sudden loss of consciousness
Antihypertensive	Alpha-2 agonist	Clonidine	Yes	0.1 mg QHS	0.1–0.4 mg/day divided	Standard + BP monitoring	Sinus bradycardia, AV block, withdrawal HTN
Antihypertensive	Beta blocker	Propranolol	Yes	Varies	Varies	Standard	Depressed myocardial contractility; Contraindicated with asthma, may mask symptoms of hypoglycemia

(continued)

Class	Subclass	Name	Generic?	Suggested starting dose for ID/DD	Effective range	Labs/studies	Serious S/E	Notes
Antipsychotic	FGA	Chlorpromazine	Yes	25 mg QHS	200–400 mg/day divided doses	Antipsychotic workup + AIMS testing	NMS, agranulocytosis, seizures, TD, QTc prolongation, black box warning (dementia-related psychosis)	
Antipsychotic	FGA	Fluphenazine	Yes	0.5 mg	0.5–40 mg/day	Antipsychotic workup + AIMS testing	NMS, agranulocytosis, jaundice, seizures, TD, QTc prolongation, black box warning (dementia-related psychosis)	
Antipsychotic	FGA	Haloperidol	Yes	0.5 mg bedtime	1–20 mg/day	Antipsychotic workup + AIMS testing	NMS, agranulocytosis, jaundice, seizures, TD, QTc prolongation, black box warning (dementia-related psychosis)	

Antipsychotic	FGA	Loxapine	Yes	10 mg BID	60–100 mg/day divided	Antipsychotic workup + AIMS testing	NMS, seizures, TD, QTc prolongation, black box warning (dementia-related psychosis)	
Antipsychotic	FGA	Perphenazine	Yes	2 mg TID	12–24 mg/day divided	Antipsychotic workup + AIMS testing	NMS, seizures, TD, jaundice, agranulocytosis, black box warning (dementia-related psychosis)	
Antipsychotic	FGA	Brexpiprazole	No	0.5 mg	2–4 mg/day	Antipsychotic workup + AIMS testing	Black box warning (SI) (dementia-related psychosis), NMS, agranulocytosis, seizures, TD	
Antipsychotic	SGA	Aripiprazole	Yes	1 mg qd	5–30 mg/day	Antipsychotic workup + AIMS testing	NMS, seizures, TD, QTc prolongation	
Antipsychotic	SGA	Asenapine	No	5 mg BID	10–20 mg/day	Antipsychotic Workup + AIMS testing	NMS, seizures, TD, QTc prolongation, black box warning (dementia-related psychosis)	May not eat or drink for 20 min after administration

(continued)

Class	Subclass	Name	Generic?	Suggested starting dose for ID/DD	Effective range	Labs/studies	Serious S/E	Notes
Antipsychotic	SGA	Clozapine	Yes	12.5 mg	300–900 mg/day divided	Antipsychotic workup + clozapine registry + AIMS testing	Agranulocytosis, ketoacidosis, PE, myocarditis, NMS, seizures, TD, QTc prolongation, black box warning (dementia-related psychosis)	Caution with missed dosing
Antipsychotic	SGA	Iloperidone	No	1 mg BID	32 mg/day	Antipsychotic workup + AIMS testing	NMS, seizures, TD, QTc prolongation, black box warning (dementia-related psychosis)	
Antipsychotic	SGA	Lurasidone	No	40 mg	40–80 mg/day	Antipsychotic workup + AIMS testing	NMS, seizures, TD, QTc prolongation, black box warning (dementia-related psychosis)	Take with food (at least 350 calories)

Antipsychotic	SGA	Olanzapine	Yes	2.5 mg QHS	5–20 mg/day	Antipsychotic workup + AIMS testing	NMS, seizures, TD, QTc prolongation, black box warning (dementia-related psychosis)	Contraindicated with parenteral benzodiazepine use
Antipsychotic	SGA	Paliperidone	Yes	3 mg	6 mg/day	Antipsychotic workup + AIMS testing	NMS, seizures, TD, QTc prolongation, black box warning (dementia-related psychosis)	
Antipsychotic	SGA	Quetiapine	Yes	12.5 mg QHS	400–800 mg/day divided	Antipsychotic workup + AIMS testing	NMS, seizures, TD, QTc prolongation, black box warning (dementia-related psychosis)	
Antipsychotic	SGA	Risperidone	Yes	0.5 mg qhs		Antipsychotic workup + AIMS testing	NMS, seizures, TD, QTc prolongation, black box warning (dementia-related psychosis)	

(continued)

Class	Subclass	Name	Generic?	Suggested starting dose for ID/DD	Effective range	Labs/studies	Serious S/E	Notes
Antipsychotic	SGA	Ziprasidone	Yes	20 mg BID	40–200 mg/day divided	Antipsychotic workup + AIMS testing	NMS, seizures, TD, QTc Prolongation, Black Box Warning (Dementia-Related Psychosis)	
Anxiolytic	5HT1a partial agonist	Buspirone	Yes	5 mg BID	20–40 mg/day	Standard	Cardiac abnormalities	
Anxiolytic	Antihistamine	Hydroxyzine	Yes	10 mg	10–100 mg/day divided	Standard	Convulsions, cardiac abnormalities, bronchodilation, respiratory depression	
Anxiolytic	Benzodiazepine	Alprazolam	Yes	No recommendation	NR	Standard	Cognitive impairment/ disorientation/ disinhibition	Avoid use in ID/DD population
Anxiolytic	Benzodiazepine	Chlordiazepoxide	Yes	No recommendation	NR	Standard	Cognitive impairment/ disorientation/ disinhibition	Avoid use in ID/DD population
Anxiolytic	Benzodiazepine	Clonazepam	Yes	No recommendation	NR	Standard	Cognitive impairment/ disorientation/ disinhibition	Avoid use in ID/DD population

Anxiolytic	Benzodiazepine	Clorazepate	Yes	No recommendation	NR	Standard	Cognitive impairment/ disorientation/ disinhibition	Avoid use in ID/DD population
Anxiolytic	Benzodiazepine	Diazepam	Yes	No recommendation	NR	Standard	Cognitive impairment/ disorientation/ disinhibition	Avoid use in ID/DD population
Anxiolytic	Benzodiazepine	Loflazepate	No	No recommendation	NR	Standard	Cognitive impairment/ disorientation/ disinhibition	Avoid use in ID/DD population
Anxiolytic	Benzodiazepine	Lorazepam	Yes	No recommendation	NR	Standard	Cognitive impairment/ disorientation/ disinhibition	Avoid use in ID/DD population
Anxiolytic	Benzodiazepine	Oxazepam	Yes	No recommendation	NR	Standard	Cognitive impairment/ disorientation/ disinhibition	Avoid use in ID/DD population
Cognitive enhancer	Cholinesterase inhibitor	Donepezil	Yes	5 mg	5–10 mg/day	Standard	Seizures, syncope	
Cognitive enhancer	Cholinesterase inhibitor	Galantamine	Yes	4 mg BID	8–24 mg/day divided	Standard	Seizures, syncope	
Cognitive enhancer	Cholinesterase inhibitor	Rivastigmine	Yes	1.5 mg BID	6–12 mg/day divided	Standard	Seizures, syncope	
Cognitive enhancer	NMDA receptor antagonist	Memantine	Yes	5 mg	20 mg/day divided	Standard	Seizures	

(continued)

Class	Subclass	Name	Generic?	Suggested starting dose for ID/DD	Effective range	Labs/studies	Serious S/E	Notes
Folate	Medical food	Methylfolate (l)	No	7.5 mg	7.5–15 mg/day	Standard + folate/ homocysteine monitoring	SI	Consider genotype test for MTHFR T or MTHFD1 A alleles
Hypnotic	Benzodiazepine	Estazolam	Yes	No recommendation	NR	Standard	Cognitive impairment/ disorientation/ disinhibition	Avoid use in ID/DD population
Hypnotic	Benzodiazepine	Flunitrazepam	No	No recommendation	NR	Standard	Cognitive impairment/ disorientation/ disinhibition	Avoid use in ID/DD population
Hypnotic	Benzodiazepine	Flurazepam	Yes	No recommendation	NR	Standard	Cognitive impairment/ disorientation/ disinhibition	Avoid use in ID/DD population
Hypnotic	Benzodiazepine	Midazolam	Yes	No recommendation	NR	Standard	Cognitive impairment/ disorientation/ disinhibition	Avoid use in ID/DD population
Hypnotic	Benzodiazepine	Quazepam	No	No recommendation	NR	Standard	Cognitive impairment/ disorientation/ disinhibition	Avoid use in ID/DD population

Hypnotic	Benzodiazepine	Temazepam	Yes	No recommendation	NR	Standard	Cognitive impairment/disorientation/disinhibition	Avoid use in ID/DD population
Hypnotic	Benzodiazepine	Triazolam	Yes	No recommendation	NR	Standard	Cognitive impairment/disorientation/disinhibition	Avoid use in ID/DD population
Hypnotic	Melatonin 1/2 receptor agonist	Ramelteon	No	8 mg OHS	8–160 mg/day	Standard	Respiratory Depression	
Hypnotic	Non-benzodiazepine	Eszopiclone	Yes	No recommendation	NR	Standard	Cognitive impairment/disorientation/disinhibition	Avoid use in ID/DD population
Hypnotic	Non-benzodiazepine	Zaleplon	Yes	No recommendation	NR	Standard	Cognitive impairment/disorientation/disinhibition	Avoid use in ID/DD population
Hypnotic	Non-benzodiazepine	Zolpidem	Yes	No recommendation	NR	Standard	Cognitive impairment/disorientation/disinhibition	Avoid use in ID/DD population
Hypnotic	Non-Benzodiazepine	Zopiclone	No	No recommendation	NR	Standard	Cognitive impairment/disorientation/disinhibition	Avoid use in ID/DD population

(continued)

Class	Subclass	Name	Generic?	Suggested starting dose for ID/DD	Effective range	Labs/studies	Serious S/E	Notes
Mood stabilizer	Anticonvulsant	Carbamazepine	Yes	Varies	Varies	Extensive	Aplastic anemia, agranulocytosis, SJS, SIADH	Psychiatrist/ neurologist oversight recommended
Mood Stabilizer	Anticonvulsant	Lamotrigine	Yes	Varies	Varies	Extensive	SJS; TEN, blood dyscrasias, aseptic meningitis, withdrawal seizures, SI	Psychiatrist/ neurologist oversight recommended
Mood Stabilizer	Anticonvulsant	Oxcarbazepine	Yes	Varies	Varies	Extensive	Hyponatremia, SI	Psychiatrist/ neurologist oversight recommended
Mood Stabilizer	Anticonvulsant	Valproate	Yes	Varies	Varies	Extensive	Hepatotoxicity, pancreatitis, SI	Psychiatrist/ neurologist oversight recommended
Mood Stabilizer		Lithium	Yes	Varies	Varies	Extensive	Li toxicity, interstitial nephritis, nephrogenic DI, cardiac abnormalities, pseudotumor cerebri, seizure	Psychiatrist/ neurologist oversight recommended

Pseudobulbar affect	NMDA receptor antagonist	Dextromethorphan	No	20 mg	40 mg/day divided	Standard	Immune-mediated thrombocytopenia, hepatotoxicity, QTc prolongation SI
Smoking cessation treatment		Varenicline	No	0.5 mg	2 mg/day divided	Standard	SI
Synthetic hormone	Thyroid hormone	Triiodothyronine	Yes	25 mcg	25–50 mcg/day	Standard + TSH monitoring	Angina pectoris, Shock, CHF
Wake-promoting	DRI	Modafinil	Yes	100 mg	100–200 mg/day	Standard	EKG changes, SI, SJS, angioedema, anaphylaxis
Wake-promoting		Armodafinil	Yes	150 mg/day	150–250 mg/day	Standard + EKG	Ischemic changes with cardiac abnormalities
OTC	Vitamin	Vitamin D3	OTC		600 IU		
OTC	Vitamin	Vitamin E	OTC		1000 IU		
OTC	Supplement	DHA/EPA	OTC		1.3–2.7 g/2000cals		
OTC	Mineral	Magnesium	OTC		400 mg		
OTC	Vitamin	Folate	OTC		400mcg–600mcg		
OTC	Mineral	Zinc	OTC		11 mg Male 8 mg Female		
OTC	Supplement	Melatonin	OTC		3–10 mg		
OTC	Vitamin	Vitamin B6	OTC		1.3 mg		
OTC	Vitamin	Vitamin B12	OTC		2.4mcg		

Chart adapted from [3–7]

References

1. Fletcher RJ, Barnhill J, Cooper SA. DM-ID-2: diagnostic manual-intellectual disability: a textbook of diagnosis of mental disorders in persons with intellectual disability. Washington D.C.: National Assn for the Dually Diagnosed Press; 2016.
2. Gentile JP, Gillig PM, editors. Psychiatry of intellectual disability: a practical manual. Hoboken: John Wiley & Sons; 2012.
3. Stahl SM, Stahl SM. Stahl's essential psychopharmacology: neuroscientific basis and practical applications. Cambridge: Cambridge university press; 2013.
4. Stern TA, et al. Massachusetts General Hospital psychopharmacology and neurotherapeutics e-book. London: Elsevier Health Sciences; 2015.
5. Stahl SM. The prescriber's guide. Cambridge: Cambridge University Press; 2011.
6. Jenkins JA, Kontos N. The Maudsley prescribing guidelines in psychiatry. J Clin Psychiatry. 2016;77(4):469.
7. Puzantian T, Balt S. The Carlat psychiatry report medication fact book for psychiatric practice: 2nd edition. Newburyport: Carlat Publishing; 2014.

Chapter 12
Psychotherapy

Julie P. Gentile and Allison E. Cowan

Introduction

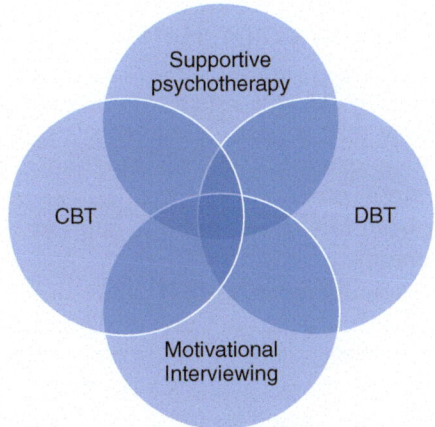

While some clinicians thought that patients with ID could not benefit from treatment with psychotherapy, others considered them protected from developing mental illnesses,

J. P. Gentile (✉) · A. E. Cowan
Department of Psychiatry, Wright State University,
Dayton, OH, USA
e-mail: julie.gentile@wright.edu; Allison.cowan@wright.edu

© Springer Nature Switzerland AG 2019   151
J. P. Gentile et al. (eds.), *Guide to Intellectual Disabilities*,
https://doi.org/10.1007/978-3-030-04456-5_12

believing that the diagnosis of ID protected individuals from developing a mental disorder because their cognitive disabilities would prevent them from experiencing emotional discord or affect [1]. It also was a widely held belief that this population did not possess the necessary skills to actively participate in the process of psychotherapy due to their diminished ability to use abstract reasoning. It was assumed that this meant that the patient did not possess the skills needed to examine their own behaviors or actions, explore potential antecedents, or to understand the benefits of making positive change.

Issues in Psychotherapy Related to ID

- Individuals with ID will experience many transitions in their lives that may trigger feelings of stress or loss [2].
  - Graduating from educational programs, transitioning from school programs to occupational settings, and moving from family settings into supported residential environments.
  - As adults, individuals with ID may desire a level of independence which is not practically possible.
- Internalized stigma regarding a diagnosis of ID: Individuals with mild ID may be particularly susceptible because they tend to have an increased awareness and understanding of their disability.
- Dependency: Most individuals with ID have a necessary dependency on family and caregivers and subsequently experience failure at a higher rate. They also often find themselves in situations in which they have little or no choice. "Learned helplessness" often develops as a reaction to this chronic sense of failure, as individuals perceive themselves to be powerless to make desired changes in their life and often feel it is futile to try.
- Reframing events with an emphasis on the situations where the individual acted in a competent way or reframing negative events as possibilities to practice new coping

skills will benefit the patient [3]. Additionally, using role-play teaches 'scripts' to use in real-life situations and increases likelihood that these new behaviors will be put into practice.

Barriers to Treatment

- Patients with ID typically are not self-referred. Most often, they are brought to treatment by a concerned care provider who seeks assistance because of some form of maladaptive behavior exhibited by the individual. The referral itself is a sensitive matter, as the individual may not see the identified issue as a problem.
- In some cases, the referral may be viewed as a punishment or consequence, and there may be confusion about the purpose of mental health services.

Lack of Understanding of Purpose of Mental Health Treatment

- It is important for the psychotherapist to spend time educating the patient about the purpose of mental health treatment. If the patient was not self-referred, they may need reassurance that they are not being punished and that the clinician is there to support them versus acting as an extension of the multidisciplinary team or referral source. Providing education regarding the purpose of therapy, the role of both the patient and the therapist, and what will occur during a typical session can dramatically enhance participation and satisfaction with mental health services and is a critical component of the therapeutic process.
- Confidentiality is the cornerstone of psychotherapy. Without the promise of confidentiality, patients would not share their inner world. Individuals with ID have the same need for confidentiality as the general population and may

withhold information out of fear of confidentiality breaches. This issue is further complicated by the fact that the psychotherapist often does need collateral information from care providers, as individuals with ID are often poor historians and may not accurately report current stressors and problems that should be addressed in treatment. The care providers can also help ensure that treatment recommendations are followed, such as completion of the homework that is assigned during sessions.

Check for Understanding

- It is important for the psychotherapist to explore the patient's degree of understanding and to ensure that the individual feels comfortable alerting the therapist if/when information is presented in a way that is confusing or unclear.
- Establish that the cognitive deficit is a legitimate and neutral topic for discussion and exploration from the beginning so that issues regarding communication can be negotiated and addressed openly.
- During sessions, it is important to explore and assess how the person describes feelings and to provide opportunities to express them. However, before this can occur the individual must have the ability to recognize and identify their emotions. The ability to identify and label feelings provides a sense of control and comfort that can increase a patient's capacity to manage emotions. It is impossible to process emotions and understand the connection between thoughts, feelings, and behaviors without the ability to first identify them. Emotions are not problems; they are signals.

Teaching the Patient to Label Feeling States

- Use of pictorial representations of faces to facilitate a patient's identification of emotions

- Use of journaling, often a useful outlet for those patients with this capacity
- Use of picture journaling can substitute for writing, by drawing or putting pictures in a journal
- Expression through music can be an excellent outlet for patients to describe their emotions

Issues Relating to Learning and Memory: Augmenting with Activities

- When working with individuals with ID, it is important to adjust the complexity of one's techniques to match the patient's level of cognitive development and to augment these techniques with activities in order to add depth to change and learning.
- These activities can include art therapy, role-play, and therapeutic games. See Table 12.1 for psychodrama techniques.

TABLE 12.1 Frequently utilized psychodrama techniques

Doubling	During role play group members share their view of the identified protagonist. The double acts as an inner voice and reflection of the protagonist.
Role reversal	The protagonist is asked to exchange roles with another person. This enables patients to view themselves from another point of view.
Soliloquizing	The protagonist to shares their most intimate thoughts about a crucial situation in their life without addressing other members of the group.
Future-projection	The protagonist projects himself into his future life.
The mirror	This technique allows the protagonist to step out of the scene and to observe someone else enacting his/her role. The protagonist can then see him/herself as others see him/her.

Adapted from reference Dayton [4]. Pages 26, 34, 35, 71

- Repetition is essential, as repeated review and practice of skills that are learned in session helps to facilitate internalization of the material presented. If the patient has a short attention span, it may be necessary to break down interventions into smaller pieces and utilize shorter session length.

Memory Aids

- The use of coping skill cards or stories can be immeasurably helpful with this, as they provide the necessary cues for the implementation of strategies or techniques; these can be easily carried in a wallet or a pocket, so they are accessible when needed in the moment.
- Laminated coping skill cards should be small, so that they can be easily carried around and accessed between sessions as needed.
- Strategies should be written in positive language that is individualized and geared to the patient's level of understanding. Pictures are often very helpful, particularly with individuals who have minimal reading skills.
- Cards should focus on one issue and should be very specific. For example, if the person wants to talk to 'someone' as a coping strategy, the card should include the designated support person's name and phone number.

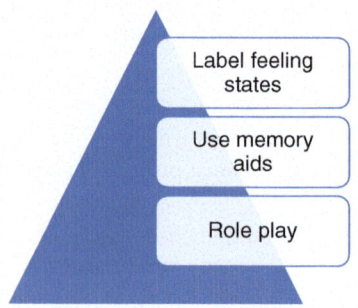

Motivational Interviewing

Motivational interviewing (MI) is a counseling approach developed by Miller and Rollnick [5] based on the theory that patients enter psychotherapy with varying levels of acceptance of their challenging behaviors and varying amounts of motivation to change them [6]. MI targets the conflicted feelings individuals often experience when thinking about making changes, with the psychotherapist working to help the patient identify, explore, and resolve ambivalence.

In order to accomplish these objectives, there are four basic techniques that clinicians use in session to help a patient gain insight into the person's problems and to increase motivation to make positive changes.

- *Open-ended questions* are used to help facilitate the flow of communication in order to create forward momentum.
- *Affirmations* are used to help restructure the patient's view of him or herself and their ability to make changes.
- *Reflective listening* is used to help the patient feel that the psychotherapist understands their point of view, as well as to help resolve ambivalence by guiding the patient to explore how the current behavior is impacting their overall quality of life and the benefits of making positive change.
- *Summaries* are a form of reflective listening that reviews what has occurred in the session. It is used to draw attention to both sides of the ambivalence the patient is experiencing while promoting the development of discrepancy through careful selection of what information is included or excluded.

MI Adapted for ID

- Take a more directive approach, helping the patient to identify and express feelings regarding the possibility of change.

- To address any barriers related to communication issues, clinicians should consider utilization of role-playing, visual prompts, pictures, therapeutic games, and activities to help facilitate the patient's involvement.

Cognitive Behavioral Therapy

Cognitive behavioral therapy (CBT) is an evidence-based and action-oriented form of psychotherapy that is based on the theory that faulty thinking patterns and the beliefs that underlie such thinking cause both maladaptive behavior and negative emotions. See Table 12.2 for adapted CBT techniques.

CBT Adapted for ID

- It may be difficult for patient with ID to identify the abstract concepts, such as thought distortions, which are central component of CBT.
- Increase the number of sessions to allow treatment to progress at a slower rate.
- Repetition of the involved components will help facilitate internalization of the necessary skills.
- Elicit the participation of involved care providers, as they can help the patient recognize and identify when the patient is experiencing cognitive distortions.
- Care providers can assist with the completion of homework assignments between sessions, such as documentation in a diary or role-play.

Dialectical Behavior Therapy

If a patient with ID is diagnosed with certain personality disorders, particularly borderline personality disorder (BPD), utilization of an evidence-based model of treatment such as

TABLE 12.2 Cognitive behavior therapy techniques

Socratic questioning	Questions that challenge the patients underlying (typically unhealthy) beliefs about themselves.
Guided discovery	This involves gentle questioning about problems designed to help the patient identify dysfunctional thinking patterns that contribute to ongoing problems or that exacerbate existing ones.
ABC model (Antecedent, Behavior, Consequence)	Use of the ABC model to help patients identify and label the connections between an activating event, their interpretation of the event, the beliefs or thoughts that occur when the event happens, and the consequences - which are the emotions and actions that are triggered by the beliefs. Once this is accomplished, the clinician can help the patient learn to objectively test whether the belief is justified or is based on erroneous assumptions.
Chain Analysis	Use of chain analysis can help a person understand the function of a particular behavior by identifying all the factors that led up to it. The individual is able to identify the situation that occurred, their subsequent responses, and all of the thoughts and feelings that occurred just prior to the behavior. Doing this can increase the individual's ability to intervene early on and prevent the behavior or feeling from occurring.
Modeling	This allows the patient and clinician to engage in role-play of different situations.
Journaling	In CBT, individuals are encouraged to keep a diary documenting their thoughts/feelings/reactions to demonstrate positive and negative consequences to behavior.

Adapted from reference Beck et al. [7]. Pages 10–12, 56, 65, 67, 110, 137, 139

dialectical behavior therapy (DBT) is appropriate and can easily be adapted to meet the needs of the individual [8]. The fact that DBT is a structured, skill-based approach makes it a particularly good fit for ID; efficacy of treatment is improved when the focus is on building replacement skills rather than merely attempting to eliminate problematic behaviors [9]. DBT was developed by Linehan [10] on the premise that the combination of exposure to an invalidating environment, along with unknown biological factions, contributes to the development of affective instability as evidenced by abnormal reactions to emotional stimulation [11, 12]. It combines four different components: CBT, dialectics, mindfulness, and validation.

DBT Adapted for ID

- It may be necessary to shorten group sessions to approximately 30–60 min and increase the frequency of group work to twice a week.
- Match the patients' cognitive needs, as well as allow for increased opportunities to practice and generalize learned skills.
- Simplify how information is presented, such as using concrete language and pictures or illustrations on homework and diary cards.
- The concepts will need to be simplified in order to increase comprehension and ability to implement skills learned.
- The use of handouts should be modified so that the language utilized matches the person's level of cognitive ability.
- Use of pictures may also be helpful to aid in the internalization of the concepts presented.
- The psychotherapist should increase the activities that are used, such as therapeutic games, role-play, etc.
- Collaborate with involved caregivers.

Supportive Psychotherapy

Supportive psychotherapy (SP) is an interactive approach, based on a model of conversation rather than silent listening, as the therapist actively engages with the patient [13]. At the core of SP is belief that the positive and supportive relationship developed between the patient and psychotherapist can serve to reinforce and repair deficits in the person's self-structure resulting from inadequate early parenting. The psychotherapist assumes an intensely empathetic introspective stance with the patient, nurturing positive transference and using it to further strengthen the relationship [11, 14, 15].

SP Adapted for ID

- Utilize a more directive and supportive approach that utilizes techniques such as suggestion, persuasion and reassurance.
- Inclusion of advocacy for patients and encouragement of involvement of concerned others.
- Simplify the interventions that are used; they should be divided into smaller units.
- Expect a longer length of treatment to allow for repetition of learned skills to facilitate retention and generalization [16].
- Augment these techniques with activities, in order to deepen change and learning. Activities could include therapeutic games, drawings, role-plays, etc.

Group Therapy

Participation in group therapy provides an opportunity to address problems with the assistance and support of other persons who have common issues and goals [17]. This results in a sense of universality, as patients come to realize that they are not alone in the struggles they are facing. In addition, there is immense benefit in witnessing the resourcefulness of group members who are in similar situations, as it provides participants with a sense of reassurance and hope in their own recovery. Ideally, the group process also can provide a safe forum to learn and practice new behaviors, without the fear of failure. The benefits of group therapy can include:

- Improved interpersonal relationships
- Improved ability to effectively utilize problem-solving skills
- Improved ability to appropriately and effectively communicate wants and needs to others
- Improved ability to manage symptoms of mental illness and stress
- Improved self-esteem and acceptance of ID

Group Therapy Adapted for ID

Studies indicate that the interactive behavioral therapy (IBT) model is the most effective with individuals with ID [18]. IBT was specifically designed for use with individuals who have some form of cognitive disability and incorporates action-based techniques that are drawn from the field of psychodrama. It is theorized that engaging the patient behaviorally, emotionally, as well as verbally enhances the patient's ability to benefit from the treatment provided.

IBT group sessions are structured into four stages: (1) an orientation stage, (2) a warm up and sharing stage, (3) an enactment stage, and (4) an affirmation stage.

- Orientation stage: facilitators work to shape good interpersonal behavior (having members repeat what was said to them, ensuring that individuals turn toward the person who is speaking, and acknowledge what was said, and/or in some way participate in the group process through interaction).
- Warm up and sharing stage: participants set agenda items and share what issue they would like to address during the

session; the group selects an issue and a protagonist around whose problems the group therapy session will revolve.

- Enactment stage: facilitators guide the group to explore the identified issues, and psychodrama techniques are utilized in order to increase emotional engagement.
- Affirmation stage: each member of the group is given feedback about the strengths and gains achieved during that particular therapy session.

Clinical Pearls for Psychotherapy for Individuals with ID
- Individuals with ID can benefit from psychotherapy.
- Check for understanding frequently.
- Consider many available adapted psychotherapies.
- Shortening the length of the session may be helpful for attentional issues.

Summary

Although historically it was believed that individual with ID could not benefit from psychotherapy, research produced in the last 10–15 years has demonstrated definitively that this is not the case. It is now understood that the efficacy of treatment improves dramatically when modifications are made to traditional treatment models so that the service delivery matches the developmental and cognitive needs of the patient. There is consensus that when working with patient with ID, the following adaptations are best practices:

- Increase length of treatment to allow for needed repetition and implementation of additional treatment stages.
- Adjust complexity of the interventions provided to match the patient's developmental framework.

- Reduce the level of vocabulary, sentence structure, and length of utterance to match individual's level of understanding.
- Utilize more directive methods.
- Provide the patient with visual cues to address memory issues.
- Augment interventions with activities to deepen understanding of information presented.
- Involve care providers with the consent of the patient.

Clinical Vignette #1

Bob, a 41-year-old male with moderate ID, was referred for psychotherapy by his multidisciplinary team due to an increase in aggression and anger outbursts directed at staff and peers. Bob's medical history was significant for seizure disorder, which was well-controlled with medication; however, his legal guardian become concerned about the potential impact of drinking large quantities of caffeine, and after a consultation with Bob's primary care physician, it was recommended that all caffeine be discontinued. Bob enjoyed drinking approximately four cans of a caffeinated beverage a day, two while at work and another two in the evening. His team, following the physician's order, replaced these beverages with caffeine-free beverage (of the same brand) which resulted in behavioral outbursts and violence directed towards the staff. At the time of the initial referral, the team and guardian requested that the focus of the treatment be to decrease aggression and increase Bob's willingness to comply with staff requests. They also voiced concern regarding Bob's ability to maintain employment and his current residential placement if his aggressive behavior continued.

Upon meeting Bob, it became clear that he did not view the problem in the same light as his team. He reported that he enjoyed beverages with caffeine and could taste the difference when staff gave him alternative options. Bob felt that he was being "controlled" and that he should have the right to make his own choices about what he eats and drinks. Bob also felt that he was taken to see a psychotherapist because he was "in trouble" due to his recent aggressive behavior and shared anxiety that the psychotherapist would share his thoughts and feelings with the team (mainly around the anger he felt towards them) – which would then lead to negative consequences for him. The first goal of therapy was to work to establish a therapeutic alliance with Bob and to focus on his wants and needs. It was important to spend time educating Bob regarding the psychotherapist's role in his life and making sure that the boundaries and limitations of confidentiality were understood. The psychotherapist was very specific about what would be shared with the team and the purpose of this collaboration. Once rapport and trust were established, Bob addressed his feelings of anger and resentment and learned more acceptable ways to communicate his wants and needs to others as well as strategies to communicate his feelings.

Clinical Vignette #2
Frances is a 49-year-old female with moderate ID, who previously resided with her mother until 3 years ago at which time her mother passed away from a terminal illness. Her father had passed away 15 years before. After her mother's death, she was uprooted from the home wherein she had spent her entire life, and moved to a group home environment across town from her childhood home. Frances was an only child, with no other

family involvement, so there was no one in her life who could either take her in or assist with the transition to a new home. She struggled with the loss of her parents and with the secondary losses that occurred as a result of their death. Residential staff attempted to help her manage her feelings for approximately 1 year and finally made the referral for mental health services after her mood remained depressed regardless of their attempts to assist her in moving forward following the multiple layers of loss. Frances's grief was complicated in that she never worked through her feelings regarding her father's death and when her mother died, she found herself grieving both losses as if they had both just occurred. In psychotherapy, Frances expressed feelings of anger at her parents for leaving her and stated her belief that if she had been a "better" daughter, they would still be alive. She also shared feelings of anger and resentment regarding the fact that she was now living in a group home and had a great deal of distrust for staff. Her parents had been the only caregivers she had ever known, and she felt unable to trust that these "strangers" would take care of her. She was particularly worried that they would steal from her or harm her in some way. Frances spent the majority of her time alone in her room, looking at pictures of her parents and thinking about their deaths.

Initial therapy sessions were focused on developing the therapeutic alliance and giving Frances a safe space to express her emotional pain. Time was spent helping her process her thoughts and feelings about the loss and exploring her spiritual beliefs. Frances identified that she knew her parents were in heaven; however, she was concerned that they were "worried" about her and her adjustment to her new home. In these early sessions she exhibited multiple crying spells which lasted for several minutes, during which time she was given support and reassurance that she would be able to cope with her overwhelming feelings of grief and loss. The psychotherapist spent time providing education regarding the life cycle and normalized her parents' deaths. They explored Frances' belief that her parents made a choice to leave her and worked to restructure her thoughts about this. She was taught coping skills to utilize when feeling overwhelmed by her feelings (relaxation techniques, journaling, and use of art), and staff were enlisted to help ensure homework was completed between sessions. Frances and her psychotherapist worked together to develop a short story book about her experiences with grief and loss. The book reviewed her life with her parents, their death, her experience of grief, her initiation of psychotherapy, coping strategies she was learning in treatment, and her hopes and goals for her future. She reviewed the book on a daily basis to help normalize her experiences, cue her to utilize learned skills, and to give her hope about the possibility of recovery.

Time was spent addressing her fears regarding her new home and staff, and examining her distorted thoughts about her move. Frances identified that she was angry with the staff because she blamed them for her move and many of the secondary losses in her life, and once she understood this and was able to accept that her parents' death and her subsequent move were not anyone's fault, her feelings of anger reduced considerably. Frances began to keep a gratitude journal, which helped her realize that there were many positive things that she could enjoy about her new life. As her mood began to lift, she experienced feelings of guilt regarding her recovery and what it meant about her love for her parents. The psychotherapist provided reassurance and support and helped Frances find ways to incorporate her memories and love for her parents into her life, while also allowing herself to move forward and build a new life on her own.

Eventually Frances became more active with her housemates, was able to build close relationships with her staff, and increase her participation in recreational activities in the community. As she made progress, her mood continued to improve and psychotherapy was slowly discontinued.

References

1. Prout HT. The effectiveness of psychotherapy with persons with intellectual disabilities. Psychotherapy for individuals with intellectual disability. Kingston: NADD Press; 2011. p. 265–87.
2. Bowlby J. Attachment and loss, Vol. 1: attachment. London: Hogarth Press and Institute of Psycho-Analysis; 1969.
3. Keller EM. Poimts of intervention: facilitating the process of psychotherapy with people who have developmental disabilities. Therapy Approahces for People with Mental Retardation. 2000:27–47.
4. Dayton T. The drama within: psychodrama and experiential therapy. Deerfield: Health Communications, Inc.; 1994.
5. Miller WR, Rollnick S. Motivational interviewing: preparing people for change. New York: Guilford Press; 2002.
6. Arkowitz H, Westra H. Introduction to the special series on motivational interviewing and psychotherapy. J Clin Psychol. 2009;65:1149–55.
7. Beck AT, Rush AJ, Shaw BF, Emery G. Cognitive theory of depression. New York: The Guilford Press; 1979.
8. Charlton M, Dykstra EJ. Dialectical behavior therapy for special populations: treatment with adolescents and their Caregivers. Psychotherapy for individuals with intellectual disabilities. Kingston: NADD Press; 2011. p. 13–36.
9. Lew M. Dialectical behavior therapy for adults who have intellectual disability. Psychotherapy for individuals with intellectual disability. Kingston: NADD Press; 2011. p. 37–66.

10. Linehan MM. Cogntivie behavioral treatment of borderline personality disorder. New York: A division of Guilford Publications, Inc.; 1993.
11. Martin A. Intellectual disability, trauma and psychotherapy. J Appl Res Intellect Disabil. 2010;23(3):301.
12. Mitchell A, Clegg J, Furniss F. Exploring the meaning of trauma with adults with intellectual disabilities. J Appl Res Intellect Disabil. 2006;19:131–42.
13. Gentile JP, Jackson CS. Supportive psychotherapy with the dual diagnosis patient. Psychiatry. 2008;5(3):49–57.
14. Fernado K, Medlicott L. My shield will protect me against the ants: treatment of PTSD in a client with intellectual disability. J Intellect Develop Disabil. 2009;34(2):187–92.
15. Mevissen L, de Jongh A. PTSD and its treatment in people with intellectual disabilities: a review of the literature. Clin Psychol Rev. 2010;30(3):308–16.
16. Clute MA. Bereavement interventions for adults with intellectual disabilities: what works? Omega. 2010;61(2):163–77.
17. Davidson PW, Cain NN. Overview. Training handbook of mental disorders in individuals with intellectual disability. Kingston: NADD Press; 2006. p. 1–13.
18. Tomasulo DL, Razzam NJ. Empirical validation of IBT for clients with intellectual disabilities. The Group Psychologist. 2009;19:3.

Chapter 13
Behavioral Interventions and Supports in Preparation for and During Transitions in Life Stages

Ronne Justine Proch and Benjamin Lee Bates

Abbreviations

ABA   Applied behavior analysis
IPS   Individual placement support
PBS   Positive behavior support
SIT   Sensory integration therapy

Pharmacology is only one aspect of a patient's treatment, and although it can certainly help facilitate appropriate behavior,

R. J. Proch
Wright State University, Boonshoft School of Medicine,
Dayton, OH, USA

Wright-Patterson AFB, Department of Psychiatry,
Dayton, OH, USA
e-mail: ronne.proch@wright.edu

B. L. Bates (✉)
Registered Behavior Technician, S/OT, University of Findlay,
Department of Occupational Therapy, Fairborn, OH, USA
e-mail: batesb1@findlay.edu

© Springer Nature Switzerland AG 2019   171
J. P. Gentile et al. (eds.), *Guide to Intellectual Disabilities*,
https://doi.org/10.1007/978-3-030-04456-5_13

it cannot solely ensure a patient's success throughout life. Family involvement and collaboration with providers as well as behavioral therapies tend to lead to more positive long-term outcomes both before adulthood and after. More recently, research has shown that patients with intellectual disability (ID) seek to be understood and heard. Those patients whom are encouraged to participate in their care via self-determination and choice tend to have better overall outcomes than those who do not participate in facilitating their care plan. Below are the aspects of treatment that tend to lead to more positive long-term outcomes in patients throughout their lives [9, 11].

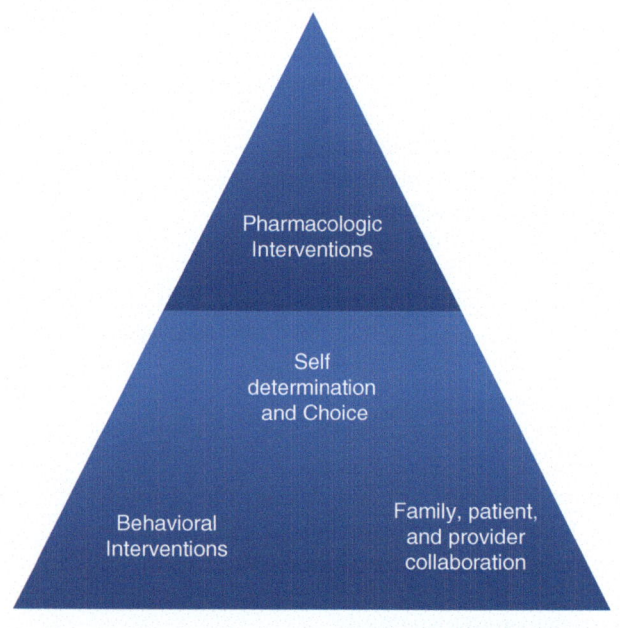

There are many well-known behavioral therapies and modalities used for patients with ID and autism spectrum disorders currently being utilized in schools, homes, and clinical settings. The majority of these theories and modalities stem from applied behavior analysis as is indicated below [1, 3, 4, 7, 8, 12].

Types of interventional therapy	
Applied behavior analysis (ABA)	Can be used in wide age range; toddler to adult
	Focuses on principles of learning; objective and goal based
	Positive reinforcement is a main tenet; decreasing negative behaviors and increasing positive behaviors
	It is initially therapist-directed but now can be directed by therapist and/or patient
	Can be used individually or in group settings
	Fosters basic skills including those mimicking the home environment
	Endorsed by multiple federal agencies including US Surgeon General in the treatment of ASD
	ABA techniques produce improvements in communication, social relationships, play, self-care, school, and employment
Early Start Denver Model	Intervention for toddlers (12–48 months) with ASD
	Therapeutic setting: clinic and/or home
	Based on ABA
	Clinical specialties involved: psychologist, behaviorist, occupational therapist, speech pathologist, early intervention specialist, and developmental pediatrician
	Contains developmental curriculum recommending that skills be taught as well as outlining teaching procedures for doing so
	Recommends parental involvement to continue therapy at home
	Found to significantly improve IQ, adaptive behavior, and autism diagnosis (more children converted to Pervasive Developmental Disorder within 2 years of implementation) in clinical trials

(*continued*)

Types of interventional therapy	
Sensory integration therapy (SIT)	Performed mostly by occupational therapists
	Focuses on participation of the patient and patient directedness
	Based on principle that one or more senses are over or under-reactive to stimulation thus driving nonpurposeful behaviors such as rocking, spinning, and hand-flapping
	Example of technique: pressure-touch; controlled sensory input to elicit adaptive motor responses
	Clinical trials have demonstrated significant positive changes in Goal Attainment Scales and decreases in stereotyped movements
Positive behavior support (PBS)	Evaluation of a challenging behavior that aids in constructing a plan for addressing the behavior
	Emerged from Applied Behavioral Analysis
	Used in the school setting most frequently
	Based on the principle that negative behaviors are reinforced by the patient's environment which make them functional by achieving some desired effect (i.e., negative actions that receive attention or objects)
	Functional behavior assessments (FBA) are used to define behaviors, identify contexts which contribute to the behavior and consequences which may perpetuate the behavior. Steps include: goal identification, information gathering, hypothesis development, support plan design, implementation, and monitoring

ABA and similar therapies are not only useful in the clinical setting. In fact, as highlighted in the Case Vignette below, cooperation from the family to continue therapy at home is essential to the overall success of the child.

Case Vignette
Jay is a 15-year-old Caucasian male diagnosed with autism at the age of 3 receiving one-on-one ABA ser-

vices in a community therapy center since he was 4 years old. He has some vocal abilities and communicates mostly through American Sign Language. Jay also exhibits tantrums (where he throws chairs and damages property) and self-injurious behaviors (SIB) such as hitting himself and throwing himself on the floor. Goals of treatment according to the family include decreasing SIB, graduating high school, and getting a part-time job afterwards. Overall, the hope is that Jay will be as independent as possible. Initially, Jay would have up to 100 discrete SIBs sometimes chained together during tantrums and had difficulty communicating his needs. Through the course of treatment, it became apparent that the family was not always enforcing ABA at home. Jay would exhibit improving behavior throughout the week and tended to decompensate over the weekend so that the process would have to start over again on Monday. This was addressed with the family, and ABA began to be applied in the home setting more frequently. His therapists now report that the frequency of his SIBs have decreased to 2–3 per day, and his goal-oriented communication has improved.

Maintaining a therapeutic environment in collaboration with medications and families correlates positively with better outcomes and long-term success. Establishing a supportive foundation is important in setting patients up for especially stressful times in their life such as transitions into adulthood as is highlighted below.

Transitioning into Adulthood: Living and Employment

- The transition into adulthood generally takes place between the ages of 16 and 25 and involves planning with the family, patient, and providers and focused on two core issues: living and employment [2, 5, 6]. Some studies suggest that families do consider quality of life in their measure of success of transition, but treatment should focus on the former, as the latter could be considered subjective.

- Future planning with families has shown to be especially important with respect to living arrangements as studies have shown that future planning tends to correlate with more independent living which most families and patients would consider most desirable. Independent living can include supports vs no supports.

- Patients not well suited for family living are often placed into group homes with supported residential settings typically decided by funding agencies [10, 13]. Lack of family planning and/or incentive to attain the highest level of independence generally results in the person with ID residing with family. This may be difficult to manage, especially during transitions or other losses or change. See figure below.

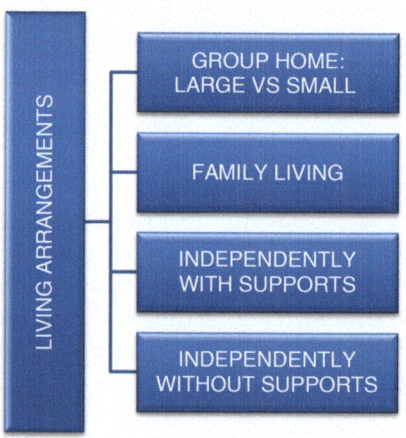

Living arrangements in adulthood contribute significantly to an individual's quality of life and long-term success, especially when self-determination and patient choice is considered and respected.

Employment

- Supported employment and Individual Placement Support (IPS) is a strategy that places adults with ID and other severe mental illnesses into competitive jobs by providing support both long term and short term to increase longevity of employment. The figure below highlights some of the tenets of IPS that are essential to fostering positive and enduring employment in patients with ID.

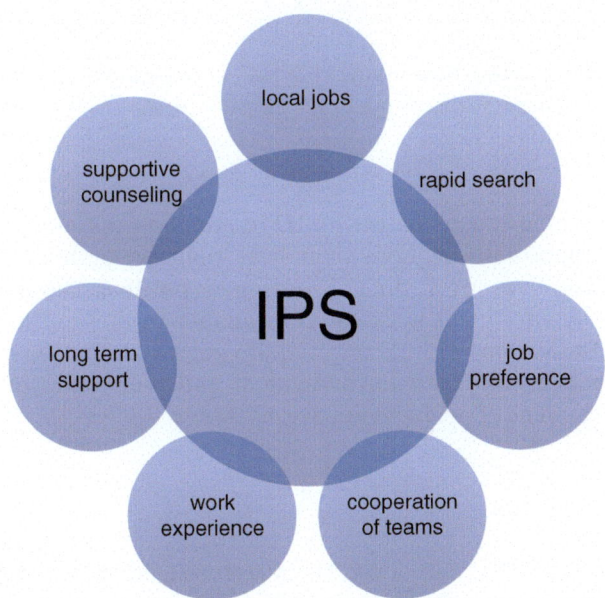

Engaging all facets of IPS as above has yielded positive results, especially for the ID and Medicaid populations. Youth participating in IPS was significantly more likely to find jobs faster and sustain employment longer according to research.

Clinical Pearls
- Early intervention is correlated with moderate positive effects in behavior long term.
- Environmental modification has been linked with improvement in quality of life.
- Self-determination and advocacy have become best practices in the field and demonstrate increases in reported quality of life.
- Future planning with families during transitional ages increases likelihood that individuals will live independently.
- Supported Employment/IPS decreases time it takes to find a job and prolongs employment.

In conclusion, patients with ID require appropriate behavioral support throughout their lives that can better ensure fulfilling lives over time. Ensuring a positive, supportive home environment is essential in quality of life and happiness. Individuals with ID may require behavioral intervention which can help both the individual and their team in the management of problem behaviors.

References

1. Ben-Itzchak E, Zachor DA. The effects of intellectual functioning and autism severity on outcome of early behavioral intervention for children with autism. Res Dev Disabil. 2007;28(3):287–303. https://doi.org/10.1016/j.ridd.2006.03.002.
2. Burke MM, et al. Individual and family correlates of community living options among adults with intellectual and developmental disabilities. Inclusion. 2017;5(4):279–92. https://doi.org/10.1352/2326-6988-5.4.279.
3. Carr EG, et al. Positive behavior support. J Posit Behav Interv. 2002;4(1):4–16. https://doi.org/10.1177/109830070200400102.
4. Dawson G, et al. Randomized, controlled trial of an intervention for toddlers with autism: the Early Start Denver

Model. Pediatrics. 2009;125(1) https://doi.org/10.1542/peds.2009-0958.

5. Henninger NA, Taylor JL. Family perspectives on a successful transition to adulthood for individuals with disabilities. Intellect Dev Disabil. 2014;52(2):98–111. https://doi.org/10.1352/1934-9556-52.2.98.

6. Kraemer BR, Blacher J. Transition for young adults with severe mental retardation: school preparation, parent expectations, and family involvement. Ment Retard. 2001;39(6):423–35. https://doi.org/10.1352/0047-6765(2001)039<0423:tfyaws>2.0.co;2.

7. Lovaas OI. Behavioral treatment and normal educational and intellectual functioning in young autistic children. J Consult Clin Psychol. 1987;55(1):3–9. https://doi.org/10.1037//0022-006x.55.1.3.

8. Pfeiffer BA, et al. Effectiveness of sensory integration interventions in children with autism Spectrum disorders: a pilot study. Am J Occup Ther. 2011;65(1):76–85. https://doi.org/10.5014/ajot.2011.09205.

9. Schalock RL, et al. Conceptualization, measurement, and application of quality of life for persons with intellectual disabilities: report of an international panel of experts. Ment Retard. 2002; 40(6):457–70. https://doi.org/10.1352/0047-6765(2002)040<0457:cmaaoq>2.0.co;2.

10. Sugai G, et al. Applying positive behavior support and functional behavioral assessment in schools. J Posit Behav Interv. 2000;2(3) https://doi.org/10.1177/109830070000200302.

11. Thompson C, et al. To be understood: transitioning to adult life for people with autism spectrum disorder. Plos One. 2018;13(3) https://doi.org/10.1371/journal.pone.0194758.

12. Virués-Ortega J. Applied behavior analytic intervention for autism in early childhood: meta-analysis, meta-regression and dose–response meta-analysis of multiple outcomes. Clin Psychol Rev. 2010;30(4):387–99. https://doi.org/10.1016/j.cpr.2010.01.008.

13. Wehman P, et al. Effect of supported employment on vocational rehabilitation outcomes of transition-age youth with intellectual and developmental disabilities: a case control study. Intellect Dev Disabil. 2014;52(4):296–310. https://doi.org/10.1352/1934-9556-52.4.296.

Chapter 14
Legal Issues Related to Intellectual Disabilities

Jeffrey Guina

Legal Definitions

All US jurisdictions (e.g., state, federal, military) define certain mental conditions for legal purposes such as civil commitment and criminal insanity. Most states have separate provisions for definitions of intellectual disability (ID), developmental disability, and "mental illness" or "mental disease" for particular purposes. Because statutes have not all been updated, even the terms "mental defect," "mental deficiency," and "mental retardation" are still seen in some statutes. Some jurisdictions use ID as exclusionary criteria for certain purposes. For example, Arizona excludes ID as grounds for civil commitment (Ariz Rev. Stat § 36–501), and Florida excludes ID and autism as grounds for an insanity defense though not for incompetence to stand trial (Florida Statutes § 916.106–916.15). These definitions can also dictate access to certain publicly funded services. Although some statutes, legal cases,

J. Guina (✉)
Center for Forensic Psychiatry, Saline, MI, USA

University of Michigan Medicine, Ann Arbor, MI, USA

Department of Psychiatry, Wright State University, Boonshoft School of Medicine, Dayton, OH, USA
e-mail: guinaj@michigan.gov

© Springer Nature Switzerland AG 2019
J. P. Gentile et al. (eds.), *Guide to Intellectual Disabilities*,
https://doi.org/10.1007/978-3-030-04456-5_14

and research studies in the academic literature may use other terminology, this chapter consistently uses "ID" for simplicity of presentation.

Case Vignette

Mr. S is a 20-year-old man charged with stalking. He has diagnoses of mild ID and autism spectrum disorder. He had significant caregiver instability growing up, experiencing abuse and neglect from his biological and various foster parents. After turning 18, he initially lived in an adult foster care home. After several months of skills training, his caseworker and his legally authorized representative worked with him, and all agreed to attempt independent living with regular support from community mental health and family. Unable to maintain employment, he supported himself with Supplemental Security Income (SSI) and financial assistance from his family, who managed his finances. After his family bought him a smartphone, he began spending most of his time on social media. The police report indicates that, for over a year, he sent several social media messages each day to acquaintances. Review of these messages revealed that they did not contain any aggressive or sexual material, but rather multiple misguided attempts to establish relationships and plan to meet socially. Despite multiple requests to stop and warnings from family, clinicians, and eventually the police, he continued to send unwanted messages. He maintained that he persisted because "we're friends." Eventually, an acquaintance pressed charges and Mr. S was arrested. His family did not take possession of the phone until he was arrested and then released on bond. He was adjudicated Competent to Stand Trial (CST) and, eventually, adjudicated not guilty by reason of insanity, resulting in commitment to a state hospital.

Federal Statutes and Supreme Court Case Law Relevant to Intellectual Disabilities (ID)

Civil Rights	
Education for All Handicapped Children Act (1975), subsumed by Individuals with Disabilities Education Act (1990)	Funds school systems that provide free public education for every child, regardless of disability
Civil Rights of Institutionalized Persons Act (1980)	Enforces the rights of individuals in medical and correctional facilities
Protection and Advocacy for Individuals with Mental Illness Act (1986)	Funds mental health patient advocacy
Americans with Disability Act (1990), subsumed by the Americans with Disabilities Amendments Act (2009)	Prohibits discrimination on the basis of disabilities in a variety of circumstances
Olmstead v. LC ex rel Zimring, 119 S.Ct. 2176 (1999)	Individuals with mental disabilities must be placed in and given access to community settings rather than being kept in institutions, when appropriate.
Civil Commitment	
O'Connor v. Donaldson, 95 S. Ct. 2486 (1975)	Individuals cannot be confined based on having a mental condition alone, without dangerousness or inability to live safely in the community with or without support
Parham v. JR and JL, 99 S.Ct. 2493 (1979)	Parents can authorize commitment of their children
Youngberg v. Romeo, 102 S.Ct 2452 (1982)	Committed patients have the right to reasonably safe conditions of confinement
Zinermon v. Burch, 110 S.Ct. 975 (1990)	Patients who lack capacity to understand why they are in the hospital should have other procedures to safeguard them for admission decisions

(continued)

(*continued*)

Heller v. Doe, 113 S.Ct. 2637 (1993)	States may have different standards and procedures for civilly committing persons with mental illness and ID
Criminal Justice	
Dusky v. US, 80 S.Ct. 788 (1960)	Defendants should be able to rationally understand criminal proceedings and assist their attorney
Jackson v. Indiana, 92 S.Ct. 1845 (1972)	Defendants who cannot be restored to competency beyond the time allowed by law require civil commitment proceedings for continued commitment
Ake v. Oklahoma, 105 S.Ct. 1087 (1985)	The state must provide at least one court-appointed forensic evaluation for insanity
Cooper v. Oklahoma, 116 S.Ct. 1373 (1996)	The standard of proof for determining incompetence to stand trial is preponderance of evidence
Atkins v. VA, 122 S.Ct. 2242 (2002)	Executing persons with ID is unconstitutional
Hall v. Florida, 134 S.Ct. 1986 (2014)	Strict intelligence score cutoffs for a diagnosis of ID for determining death penalty eligibility is unconstitutional

Civil Rights

Throughout history, persons with ID have been vulnerable to stigma, ridicule, discrimination, and abuse, sometimes by the state (e.g., ancient Sparta, medieval court jesters, Nazi Germany). Legal protection for individuals with ID is a relatively recent concept. The Americans with Disability Act (ADA) prohibits discrimination against people with ID, in a variety of circumstances including employment, housing, public services, and in public and private facilities. Protections against discrimination are particularly important for individuals with ID, who often will not advocate for themselves because of limited understanding, communication deficits, and/or a tendency to underreport their deficits/needs due to shame and stigma. Because individuals with ID tend to deny or be unaware of their disabilities, it typically falls on those around them—family, clinicians, teachers, and caregivers—to advocate for them to receive supports in matters they cannot help themselves.

The Civil Rights of Institutionalized Persons Act provides for federal interventions—via the Department of Justice—when patient rights are violated in psychiatric hospitals, developmental centers/facilities, nursing homes, and correctional facilities. The Protection and Advocacy for Individuals with Mental Illness Act provides federal funds to patient advocacy agencies employing lawyers who investigate civil rights violations. Initially, this law applied only to institutions, but the mandate has since grown to apply to the community as well. Data suggests that legal protections have led to a decrease in abuse and neglect cases, although this may also be due to a reduction in psychiatric bed availability ([6], p. 129).

Abuse/Neglect

Individuals with ID are vulnerable to abuse, neglect, and exploitation by virtue of difficulty caring and advocating for themselves, impaired judgment, and maladaptive behaviors. Often, people with ID will not report victimization because they do not know how to seek protection, have communication deficits, and/or are dependent on their abusers for basic needs. Therefore, they are often dependent on others to report suspected maltreatment/crimes. All states have mandatory abuse reporting, though there may be differences in thresholds for reporting, who is mandated to report, and which ages or conditions qualify for protective services. For example, all states require reporting for child abuse, but many jurisdictions also cover vulnerable adults such as the elderly and/or persons with developmental or physical disabilities.

Mandated reporters are immune from liability if they make a good faith effort to comply with their state's law, but those who fail to comply or make false reports can face criminal charges and/or civil liability.

Educational Rights

Educational opportunities have greatly expanded for individuals with ID, both due to legal mandates and societal awareness. The Individuals with Disabilities Education Act requires every school system in the USA, in return for federal funding, to provide free public education for everyone 3–22 years old. This requirement is regardless of the presence or severity of a disability and requires schools to provide the least restrictive environment that is appropriate for a student's needs. Many individuals with ID receive special education in segregated classrooms, while some have "mainstreamed" in integrated classrooms with varying levels of support. Modifications and accommodations may include less material to cover, different approaches to teaching, extended time for tests/assignments, simplified or shorter tests/assignments, opportunity for breaks, access to quiet spaces or resource rooms, access to word banks or technology (e.g., calculators, audiobooks, text-to-speech software), rehabilitation counseling, and/or occupational therapy.

Entitlements

Many individuals with ID qualify for government compensation or entitlements to services. The federal government has two main disability programs: Social Security Disability (SSD) and Supplemental Security Income (SSI). Although both programs are managed by the Social Security Administration, funding and qualification requirements differ. SSD is funded by the Social Security Trust Fund from payroll taxes, and eligibility is based on having a disability and having worked longer than a certain threshold (i.e., paid enough payroll taxes themselves). SSI is funded by general taxpayer funds, and eligibility is based on having a disability and having assets/income below a certain threshold (i.e., means-tested) independent of work history. For children receiving SSI, 8% have ID, less than one-third live in a household with both parents, and, on average, SSI payments account for nearly half of the family's income [16]. Because ID is a stable condition, those who are unable to sustain employment usually only ever qualify for SSI. Those with SSI often also qualify for the Supplemental Nutrition Assistance Program ("food stamps") and Medicaid (automatically, in some states), and those with SSD often also qualify for Medicare (though after a waiting period).

Community Support

With increasing emphasis on civil rights and autonomy, and the development of efficacious medications in the 1950s–1970s, mental healthcare began to shift away from mental institutionalization. Unlike psychotic and mood disorders, there are no efficacious pharmacotherapies to treat the underlying causes of ID. Nevertheless, many mental health professionals, attorneys, and organizations have advocated for deinstitutionalization of ID to prevent "warehousing" and maximize self-determination. Subsequently, many hospitals, "developmental centers," and "state schools" have downsized or closed. The emphasis of treatment has shifted from institutions to outpatient mental health clinics, community rehabilitation programs, social skills training, vocational training, family support, independent caregivers, and/or residential accommodation or group home placements. Some of these services are provided by private and nonprofit organizations, but many are government funded.

The Supreme Court ruled in *Olmstead v. LC* that, under the ADA, states must provide community placements for persons with mental disabilities when clinically appropriate, the person does not object, and "the placement can be reasonably accommodated, taking into account the resources available to the State and the needs of others with mental disabilities." Individuals with ID often require significant support to live safely, whether for their basic needs, instrumental activities of daily living (e.g., managing finances, shopping, transportation), and/or redirection and encouragement. Some people with ID live independently or semi-independently, while others require around-the-clock supervision and/or total care. Some live with loved ones who provide all the support they need, and some have Direct Support Professionals or caregivers that help them as they live alone or with housemates. Many individuals with ID are assigned caseworkers or support administrators to oversee their services and advocate for their needs.

Many communities provide opportunities for vocational or recreational activities. Employment support may involve training programs for a workplace in the general community or in segregated/sheltered "workshops" or "business services" specifically designed for individuals with ID. Developmental workshops commonly involve cleaning, mailing/packaging, gardening/farming, sewing, assembly line work, or metal/woodwork. Some people use such workshops to transition toward integrated/competitive employment in the general community, though most remain at a workshop for the rest of their working life. While workshop employees often make less than minimum wage, the structure, social opportunities, and sense of meaning that vocational activities can provide individuals with ID can be very important to their lives. For those without the ability or desire to work, who do not have access to supported vocational activities, or for whose families/caregivers require respite, developmental "day centers" often provide nonvocational activities. These can include physical activities, games, music, crafts, day trips (e.g., movies, museums), life skills training, and/or occupational therapy. Like work, these activities can provide structure, social opportunities, and a sense of meaning to the lives of those with disabilities.

Employment Rights

A large national survey found that about one-third of individuals with ID are employed, of which 26% work full time. Employment, especially in the general community, is associated with younger age, early work experience, high adaptive functioning, and less emotional/behavioral problems. Over half of employed people with ID work in competitive settings—usually in customer, retail, or food services—while 38% work in sheltered workshops [17].

The ADA requires employers to make accommodations for individuals with ID, so long as accommodations are "reasonable" in that they do not inflict an undue hardship on employers. Accommodations may include simplified assignments, opportunities for breaks, sensitivity training for co-workers, one-to-one communication with supervisors, verbal reminders, written checklists, and using pictures/diagrams instead of words. Employees must identify themselves as disabled, provide mental health documentation, and engage their employer in a process to identify and address needs. Employers can face liability if they refuse or delay this process. However, if the individual with ID is not qualified to perform essential job functions (e.g., cannot read or file alphabetically when applying for a mailroom job), employers are not required to offer or maintain employment. Unfortunately, because individuals with ID often deny their disabilities and may have difficulty strategically engaging their employers to meet their needs, some individuals with ID may require support from and advocacy with employers.

Parental Rights

Sexuality among individuals with ID is an important topic but one that at times is not openly discussed. It is important to realize that many, if not most, individuals with ID have sex and some have children. Sex can be an appropriate activity for many but can also be potentially problematic for individuals with ID due to vulnerability to exploitation, difficulties with impulsivity, limited self-protection skills (e.g., use of condoms), and pregnancy/child-rearing. About 20% of children of individuals with ID also have ID themselves ([12], pp. 522–523), which can potentially exacerbate the inherent difficulty of raising children. Most states have language that specifically refers to or encompasses ID as potential grounds for terminating parental rights [10]. While parents with ID are overrepresented in the child protective system for neglect, it is unclear if this is due to factors directly or indirectly related to ID. For example, parents with ID may be inherently more likely to neglect their children, and/or ID is associated with factors like poverty and having children with ID which are associated with neglect. Like the termination of the parental rights of other people, terminating the parental rights of individuals with ID requires due process and often principles including "best interest of the child," "least detrimental alternative," and efforts for reunification when possible [15].

Civil Competencies

Persons with ID often have difficulties making some decisions in their own best interests. They are particularly vulnerable to being influenced against their own wishes or taken advantage of financially and/or sexually. For these reasons, it is not uncommon for family members to raise the issue of competency when individuals with ID refuse a medical treatment, spend money on nonessentials while neglecting their own needs, write a will, or enter into a marriage contract (which some states prohibit or limit). Therefore, they often require supported or alternate decision-making for some or all important decisions [8]. Clinicians may sometimes be required to assess someone for decisional capacity (a clinical determination) and/or for competency (a legal determination that typically requires clinical evaluation). It is important for clinicians to be clear about whether the question at hand is for task-specific capacity/competency or global competency. Different jurisdictions have different statutes regarding civil competencies, such as competency to make medical decisions (i.e., to provide informed consent or refuse treatment), capacity to contract (i.e., to make legally binding agreements), and testamentary capacity (i.e., to make wills).

Guardianship

Guardianship is the granting of one person the legal authority and fiduciary duty to care for another person—usually a minor or disabled/incapacitated adult—and that person's property. Guardians may make decisions about finances/property (i.e., guardian of estate or conservator), health/treatment and placement (i.e., guardian of person), and/or general activities. In order to protect autonomy, courts attempt to limit guardianship to specific tasks based on the individual's functioning, but full or general guardianship is granted in some cases ([6], pp. 185–198).

When a clinician provides care for an individual with ID, it is important that they inquire about and obtain legal paperwork about guardianship. Guardian consent is required and should be obtained for treatment. Though it is not necessary, working with patients to obtain "assent" can be beneficial for improving motivation, therapeutic alliance, and treatment adherence. Conflicts can sometimes be avoided if multiple reasonable treatment options are provided to patients (e.g., two or three equally efficacious medications).

Civil Commitment

The ultimate purpose of civil commitment is to provide treatment, although by its nature it involves a court order and an involuntary element that (hopefully, temporarily) limits liberty. It is generally utilized to address illness and reduce risk of harm to oneself or others due to symptoms of that illness (though civil commitment can be used for other issues such as substance use in some jurisdictions). In the case of individuals with ID, for which medications will not result in remission as they can for psychotic and mood disorder, appropriate commitment should involve skills training, conditioning/habituation, post-hospitalization safety planning, striving to find less restrictive alternatives, and—when appropriate—the use of medications to manage symptoms and comorbid conditions.

The US Supreme Court has made several rulings in the attempt to balance autonomy and safety when making commitment determinations. *Heller v. Doe* resulted from a challenge to a Kentucky statute that specified different procedures for the civil commitment of persons with ID and those with mental illness, which is typical of many jurisdictions. For example, the standard of proof in mental illness cases was beyond a reasonable doubt, while the standard was the lower clear and convincing evidence in ID cases. Reversing lower court decisions, the Supreme Court ruled that these different standards did not violate the Fourteenth Amendment (equal protection) because, unlike mental illness, ID is "a permanent, relatively static condition," "usually well documented throughout childhood, [and] is easier to diagnose than is mental illness, which may have a sudden onset in adulthood." In *O'Connor v. Donaldson*, the Supreme Court ruled that mental illness or ID alone is insufficient for commitment. More than simply having a mental illness is required to justify civil commitment, and the state cannot commit individuals who are able to safely live independently or with the support of others without that justification (e.g., dangerousness). In *Parham v. JR and JL*, the Supreme Court ruled that parents can authorize commitment of their children if a physician accepts the admission, thus bypassing the court proceedings typically required for the involuntary commitment of competent adults. In *Zinermon v. Burch*, the Supreme Court ruled that incompetent patients cannot voluntarily commit themselves. Therefore, clinicians are required to assess decisional capacity before accepting voluntary admission. *Youngberg v. Romeo* resulted from a case involving a person with profound ID who had been injured on multiple occasions while being physically restrained during involuntary hospitalization. The Supreme Court ruled that committed patients have the right, under the Fourteenth Amendment (due process), to reasonably safe conditions of confinement, freedom from unreasonable bodily restraints, and minimally adequate skills training.

Most jurisdictions have statutes prohibiting involuntary hospitalization without consideration for a less restrictive alternative that could provide appropriate care/support. Different jurisdictions have different requirements for making a determination of a least restrictive alternative. For example, Ohio statute requires courts to order the least restrictive alternative treatment plan that is "available and consistent with treatment goals" while considering diagnosis, prognosis, and patient preference (Ohio Revised Code § 5122.15[E]). Less restrictive alternatives to involuntary commitment on a locked hospital unit include hospitals with less restriction of movement, supervised residential placements (e.g., crisis housing, nursing homes, adult foster care, group homes, halfway houses, or supervision by responsible relatives), and living with family or independently with varying stipulations (e.g., conditional release, outpatient commitment, regular monitoring for treatment adherence, and substance avoidance). Even outside of hospitals, there are varying degrees of care that may be available including partial hospitalization, intensive outpatient programs, assertive community treatment, case management, and mandated frequency of various types of treatment appointments.

Criminal Justice

By virtue of having difficulty thinking, understanding, and communicating, individuals with ID often have difficulty regulating their mood and behavior. This can be further exacerbated by past or present mistreatment, for example, learned behavior or trauma-related irritability following exposure to violence, or lack of social skills and interpersonal awareness due to neglect/deprivation. With proper supervision, support, training, and treatment, problematic behaviors can often be redirected and/or discussed in the context of understanding behavior as a form of communicating distress. Without (and sometimes even with) supervision, individuals with ID sometimes commit crimes.

Despite comprising 2–3% of the population, individuals with ID comprise 4–10% of the prison population ([13], p. 1). A simple explanation of this overrepresentation may be that individuals with ID simply engage in more criminal behavior. This may be directly due to risks related to ID (e.g., mood dysregulation, impaired judgment, suggestibility) or indirectly due to more vulnerability to trauma and poverty. For example, research suggests that 31% of sexual offenders have a developmental disability, which is comparably lower than rates for paraphilias (65%), mood disorders (56%), substance use disorders (55%), and personality disorders (47%) but higher than rates for psychotic disorders (16%) and dementia (10%) ([1], pp. 193–208). However, research has suggested that many sexual offenders with ID have a history of sexual victimization, and being an offender is linked with earlier victimization [5]. Other potential explanations for individuals with ID being overrepresented in the criminal justice system include increased vulnerability to arrest, less access to effective defense attorneys, incompetence to waive Miranda rights, giving ambiguous responses to police interrogation, and/or false confessions. In a survey of individuals with ID, 68% reported believing a police officer would protect them if arrested, 58% would talk to the police before talking to a lawyer, and 38% thought they could be arrested simply for having a disability ([13], p. 12).

In part because of an increased vulnerability to criminal justice system involvement and increased vulnerability to victimization while incarcerated (e.g., extortion, theft, assault, rape), many advocates and policy makers have developed strategies for diversion. Many jurisdictions have established programs spanning law enforcement, clinical, court, and corrections systems to divert individuals with ID who would be better served elsewhere toward treatment rather than incarceration. Through community mental health treatment, police training, and providing courts with alternative options to incarceration, diversion can be highly successful. Research has demonstrated that diversion can improve mental health outcomes, reduce criminal recidivism, improve public safety, and reduce public costs [3, 4, 7, 9, 11, 14].

Competency to Stand Trial

In *Dusky v. US*, the Supreme Court ruled that defendants are incompetent to stand trial (IST) if they do not have a rational understanding of the proceedings or are unable to assist their attorney. Because individuals with ID inherently have difficulty thinking and understanding, they are particularly vulnerable to being IST. In fact, about 13–36% of persons with ID who are referred for a CST evaluation are found IST. This makes ID the third most common condition to result in IST, after psychotic disorders (45–65%) and mood disorders (23–37%) ([18], p. 342). It should be noted that the majority of individuals with ID are found CST. This is because the bar is relatively low to be considered CST. Though the exact language differs by jurisdiction, defendants need not have the same level of legal acumen as a lawyer but must simply be capable of learning the basics about their charges, the proceedings, and reasonably heeding their attorney's counsel as they consider their defense options. However, a common problem for individuals with ID—like with juvenile defendants—is difficulty making decisions about plea bargains as it involves weighing short-term and long-term risks and rewards. Therefore, it is particularly important that evaluations assess capacity to learn the pros and cons and to consider counsel's advice with regard to plea offers vs. going to trial. While the threshold for being CST may be considered low, the threshold for detecting IST is also low. In *Cooper v. Oklahoma*, the Supreme Court lowered the IST standard of proof from clear and convincing to preponderance of evidence, thus ensuring due process with a low threshold for detecting incompetent defendants.

When persons with ID are found IST, they are actually less likely to be restored to competency than persons with other mental disorders (i.e., found permanently IST). The restorability rate of individuals with ID found IST is 24–33% ([12], p. 162). Restoration for psychotic and mood disorders typically relies chiefly on medication to restore cognitive function, but for persons with ID, restoration primarily involves education (e.g., classes, one-on-one, videos). When assessing CST, it is important to note that prior knowledge is not required but merely the capacity to learn information. With time and repetition, a sizable minority of individuals with ID can learn and be restored to competency. It should be noted, however, that the time allotted for restoration varies depending on the jurisdiction and charges. In *Jackson v. Indiana*, the Supreme Court ruled that the length of commitment for someone found IST must not exceed the time required to determine the probability that the defendant is restorable. If restoration is not possible, indefinite commitment without due process is unconstitutional, and continued commitment requires civil commitment proceedings.

In addition to the standard forensic interview and records review, there are several tools to assess competency. The Competency Assessment for Standing Trial for Defendants with Mental Retardation (CAST-MR) is one of the few designed for ID (e.g., written at a 4th grade reading level) ([18], p. 351; [12], p. 155–156). However, it should be noted that the standard for CST is the same for all people (i.e., there is no separate CST standard for those with ID), so many would argue that tests need not be normed on individuals with ID and the evaluation/tools used should also be the same for all people.

Criminal Responsibility

Unlike CST evaluations, insanity or criminal responsibility evaluations require a retrospective assessment of the mental state of a defendant at the time of the alleged offense. This evaluation typically involves a forensic interview and records review (e.g., police reports, recordings, treatment records) but may also involve interviewing witnesses and/or performing psychological testing. In *Ake v. Oklahoma*, the Supreme Court ruled that the state must provide at least one court-appointed forensic evaluation for insanity if deemed necessary and defendants are unable to afford one themselves.

More so than for IST, the language used in insanity statutes significantly differ depending on jurisdictions. Some jurisdictions do not have insanity statutes but all that do require, at the very least, the presence of some sort of mental condition at the time of the alleged offenses. Jurisdictions may specify different combinations of cognitive (e.g., "nature and quality" and/or "wrongfulness") and volitional prongs (e.g., "capacity to conform conduct") that result from a mental condition in order to be found not guilty by reason of insanity. Several states use both cognitive and volitional prongs (e.g., Arkansas, Massachusetts, Michigan, and Oregon). The cognitive prong is a stricter standard because it focuses only on defendants' cognition about their conduct, though the understanding of this strictness may vary depending on the language used. For example, "know" is often considered stricter than "understand" or "appreciate" (as used in jurisdictions such as California, Florida, Ohio, and Texas).

Death Penalty

The public and juries tend to view offenders with ID as having less "death-worthiness" when considering potential death penalty sentencing [2]. In accordance with this line of thinking, multiple Supreme Court rulings have set limitations on sentencing individuals with ID who are found guilty of capital offenses. In *Atkins v. VA*, the Supreme Court ruled that executing individuals with ID violated the Eight Amendment (cruel and unusual punishment) based on "evolving standards of decency." Therefore, jurisdictions with the death penalty often necessitate evaluations for competency to be executed. In *Hall v. Florida*, the Supreme Court ruled that the use of strict IQ cutoffs for a diagnosis of ID in death penalty sentencing violates the Eight Amendment. This is consistent with changes between *DSM-IV-TR* and *DSM-5*, which does not have any specific IQ requirements but focuses instead on adaptive functioning (i.e., conceptual, social, practical) deficits.

Malingering/Feigning

Because a diagnosis of ID could potentially lead to financial or legal benefits (e.g., disability compensation, delaying a trial, avoiding incarceration, or execution), malingering must be a consideration in forensic settings. Unlike most other malingering, which involves overreporting and/or falsely producing symptoms, malingering ID involves feigning the absence of functioning. Structured, standardized assessments and performance validity are the "evidentiary gold standard" for determining feigned cognitive impairment. Individuals feigning cognitive deficits tend to have much lower scores on testing than those with true ID. Examiners should be aware of insufficient effort and responses that are inconsistent across tests of similar domains, inconsistent with real-life adaptive functioning, and inconsistent with typical ID. It is also important to note that, as opposed to malingerers, people with ID tend to minimize their deficits in self-report and are often particularly ashamed when they cannot correctly answer questions (or particularly proud when they can). Common intelligence quotient (IQ) tests (e.g., Wechsler Adult Intelligence Scale) and adaptive behavior tests (e.g., Adaptive Behavior Assessment System) do not have validity scales and are insufficient to detect malingering ([12], pp. 60–61). However, the Validity Indicator Profile was developed specifically to identify feigned ID and can be co-administered with other tests when malingering is suspected. There are also performance validity tests for memory that are sometimes used for suspected malingering of ID (e.g., the Test of Memory Malingering, the Fifteen-Item Test) ([6], pp. 83–84).

Conclusion

Individuals with ID have always been a part of society, though the extent of their participation in and their treatment by society has varied across cultures and time. Though statutes and case law can differ in different jurisdictions, most have sought to balance individual autonomy while protecting vulnerability among people with ID. Civil rights laws require the state to provide individuals with ID with certain services (e.g., housing, treatment, education) and to guard against discrimination and maltreatment. When individuals with ID are incompetent globally or in specific tasks, guardians can be appointed to care for people who are unable to care for themselves and are vulnerable to exploitation. When dangerous, civil commitment laws are in place to both provide involuntary treatment while protecting individuals with ID from unjustified loss of liberty. On occasions when people with ID enter the criminal justice system, most jurisdictions have protections to ensure they receive due process and are afforded forensic evaluations for CST and criminal responsibility.

Clinical Pearls
- Persons with intellectual disability are vulnerable to discrimination, victimization, and criminal justice involvement.
- Clinicians should be aware of who is covered by mandated reporting laws for abuse and neglect in their state.
- Persons with intellectual disability have many legal civil rights protections and entitlements

- Clinicians should address medicolegal issues such as decisional capacity, guardianship, and informed consent with their patients with intellectual disability.
- Jurisdictions vary based on how civil commitment, civil and criminal competencies, and criminal responsibility apply to persons with intellectual disability.
- Civil commitment based on intellectual disability alone is insufficient without dangerousness and, in many jurisdictions, without comorbid mental illness/disease.

References

1. Booth BD. Special populations: mentally disordered sexual offenders (MDSOs). In: Harrison K, editor. Managing high-risk sex offenders in the community: risk management, treatment and social responsibilities. Cullompton: Willan; 2010.
2. Boots D, Cochran J, Heide K. Capital punishment preferences for special offender populations. J Criminal Justice. 2003;31(6):553–65.
3. Case B, Steadman HJ, Dupuis SA, Morris LS. Who succeeds in jail diversion programs for persons with mental illness? A multi-site study. Behav Sci Law. 2009;27(5):661–74.
4. Cowell AJ, Hinde JM, Broner N, Aldridge AP. The impact on taxpayer costs of a jail diversion program for people with serious mental illness. Eval Program Plann. 2013;41:31–7.
5. Firth H, Balogh R, Berney T, Bretherton K, Graham S, Whibley S. Psychopathology of sexual abuse in young people with intellectual disability. J Intellect Disabil Res. 2001;45(3):244–52.
6. Gold LH, Frierson RL. The American Psychiatric Publishing textbook of forensic psychiatry. 3rd ed. Arlington: American Psychiatric Publishing; 2018.
7. Hayhurst KP, Leitner M, Davies L, Flentje R, Millar T, Jones A, King C, Donmall M, Farrell M, Fazel S, Harris R, Hickman M, Lennox C, Mayet S, Senior J, Shaw J. The effectiveness and cost-effectiveness of diversion and aftercare programmes for offenders using class A drugs: a systematic review and economic evaluation. Health Technol Assess. 2015;19(6):1–168.

8. Jameson JM, Riesen T, Polychronis S, Trader B, Mizner S, Martinis J, Hoyle D. Guardianship and the potential of supported decision making with individuals with disabilities. Res Pract Persons Severe Disabil. 2015;40(1):36–51.

9. Kane E, Evans E, Shokraneh F. Effectiveness of current policing-related mental health interventions: a systematic review. Behav Ment Health. 2017; https://doi.org/10.1002/cbm.2058.

10. Lightfoot E, LaLiberte T. The inclusion of disability as grounds for termination of parental rights in state codes. Policy Res Brief. 2006;17(2):1–11.

11. Lowder EM, Rade CB, Desmarais SL. Effectiveness of mental health courts in reducing recidivism: a meta-analysis. Psychiatr Serv. 2018;69(1):15–22.

12. Melton GB, Petrila J, Pythress NG, Slobogin C. Psychological evaluations for the courts: a handbook for mental health professionals and lawyers. 3rd ed. New York: Guilford Press; 2007.

13. Petersilia J. Doing justice? Criminal offenders with developmental disabilities. Berkeley: California Policy Research Center; 2000.

14. Pinals DA, Felthous AR. Introduction to this double issue: jail diversion and collaboration across the justice continuum. Behav Sci Law. 2017;35(5–6):375–9.

15. Rosner R. Principles & practice of forensic psychiatry. 2nd ed. New York: Oxford University Press; 2003.

16. Rupp K, Davies PS, Newcomb C, Iams H, Becker C, Mulpuru S, Ressler S, Romig K, Miller B. A profile of children with disabilities receiving SSI: highlights from the National Survey of SSI Children and Families. Soc Secur Bull. 2006;66(2):21–48.

17. Siperstein GN, Heyman M, Stokes JE. Pathways to employment: a national survey of adults with intellectual disabilities. J Vocat Rehabil. 2014;41(3):165–78.

18. Simon SI, Gold LH. The American Psychiatric Publishing textbook of forensic psychiatry. 2nd ed. Arlington: American Psychiatric Publishing; 2010.

Chapter 15
Syndromes of Intellectual Disability

Allison E. Cowan

Understanding specific syndromes of intellectual disability (ID) can be helpful in better recognizing distinct presentations as well as being aware of co-occurring psychiatric and medical comorbidities. What follows are the most common causes of ID as well as descriptions of elements of each syndrome with the caveat that there are many ill-defined and not -yet -defined syndromes of ID.

Fetal Alcohol Spectrum Disorder/Fetal Alcohol Syndrome

- Fetal alcohol spectrum disorders (FASD) are caused by in utero exposure to alcohol and can result in ID, behavioral and psychiatric complications, and specific facial features [1]. It is considered the most preventable cause of birth defects and ID. FASD has a worldwide prevalence of 7.7 per 1000 births worldwide and with the highest prevalence in Europe at 19.8 per 1000 births [2]

A. E. Cowan (✉)
Department of Psychiatry, Wright State University,
Dayton, OH, USA
e-mail: Allison.cowan@wright.edu

© Springer Nature Switzerland AG 2019
J. P. Gentile et al. (eds.), *Guide to Intellectual Disabilities*,
https://doi.org/10.1007/978-3-030-04456-5_15

- FASD is classified in the ICD-10 as congenital malformation syndrome due to known exogenous causes, not elsewhere classified
- Diagnosis of fetal alcohol syndrome (FAS) requires:
  - All three distinctive facial features (see below)
  - Growth deficits
  - Central nervous system problems, for example, low IQ, developmental delays, difficulty with social skills, or hyperactivity
- There is no safe amount of alcohol to drink in pregnancy, but some risk factors have been outlined [3]:
  - Quantity of alcohol—specifically binge drinking
  - Timing of maternal drinking—key facial features from FASD develop between gestational age of 6–9 weeks
  - Higher maternal age results in higher likelihood of having a child who is more severely affected
  - Higher number of previous pregnancies
  - Lower maternal BMI (body mass index)
- Individuals exposed to alcohol while in utero are known to have a constellation of facial features including:
  - Smooth philtrum (required for diagnosis of FAS)
  - Flat nasal bridge
  - Short distance between the inner and outer corners of the eyes, "wide-set eyes" (required for diagnosis of FAS)
  - Thin upper lip (required for diagnosis of FAS)
- Individuals with FASD are also more likely to have medical conditions such as:
  - Vision impairments
  - Hearing impairments
  - Sleep problems as an infant
  - Cardiac, renal, and skeletal abnormalities [4]
- Psychiatric and behavioral comorbidities:
  - Over 80% of children with heavy prenatal alcohol exposure met criteria for a psychiatric disorder [5].
    - 61% have diagnosis of mood disorder.
  - Attention Deficit Hyperactivity Disorder (ADHD) is noted to be comorbid in upward of 50% of individuals with FASD [6].

- Difficulty with adaptive behavior including opposi-
  tional defiant behavior [7].
- Individuals in a sample FASD population were found to
  be:
  - More likely to have disrupted school experience
  - More likely to have legal involvement
  - More likely to exhibit inappropriate sexual behaviors
  - And more likely to have alcohol and drug misuse
    [8]
- Treatment of FASD
  - Early identification of FASD decreases the chances of
    negative outcomes [8].
  - Treatment of co-occurring psychiatric conditions includ-
    ing Oppositional Defiant Disorder, ADHD, and ID.
- *Clinical Pearl*: Verification of maternal alcohol intake is
  not necessary in diagnosing FASD.

Autism Spectrum Disorder

Autism spectrum disorder (ASD) is described as persistent
deficits in social interactions in multiple contexts and repetitive patters or behavior, interests, or activities [9].

- ASD symptoms must be present in the early developmental period, must cause clinically significant impairments,
  and are not better explained by ID or global developmental delay alone [9].
- Autism spectrum disorders are recognized to occur in 1 in
  59 children in the USA [10].
- While individuals with ASD do not necessarily have ID,
  individuals with ID and co-occurring ASD have considerable overlap [11].
- This diagnosis can be made on clinical criteria alone or, in
  more difficult cases, the use of standardized instruments in
  neuropsychological testing.
- 70% of children had at least one comorbid disorder, and
  41% had two or more.

- Significant co-occurring psychiatric disorders include:
  - Social anxiety disorder (29%)
  - ADHD (28%)
  - Oppositional defiant disorder (28%) [12]
- Typically, most concerning for families, caregivers, and loved ones is the incidence of self-injury with upwards of 50% of individuals with ASD exhibiting self-injury [13]. This can include head-banging, hitting oneself, or biting hands.
- "Stimming" is a term that is used by the ASD community to describe self-stimulatory behavior that is commonly repetitive movements or sounds. Common stims include flapping (flapping one's hands), rocking back and forth, humming, or repetitive use of objects.
- Differential diagnoses:
  - Normal variant of behavior
  - Stereotypic movement disorder or a tic disorder
  - Intellectual disability without ASD
  - Oppositional defiant disorder
  - Attention deficit hyperactivity disorder (ADHD)
  - Selective mutism
  - Schizophrenia
- Treatment of ASD:
  - Currently only two medications are approved by the Food and Drug Administration (FDA) for use in the treatment of autism. These medications are aripiprazole and risperidone, and they target the irritability associated with autism in children aged 5 and older (risperidone) and children aged 6–17 (aripiprazole).
  - Off-label medications include clozapine, haloperidol, and sertraline [14].
  - Other treatments include:
    - Applied behavioral analysis
    - Occupational therapy with sensory integration components
    - Speech therapy for speech delay and other language deficits
    - Family therapy
- There has been no link between vaccines and autism [15, 16].

- *Clinical Pearl*: Consider occupational therapy with a sensory evaluation and a thorough medical workup when treating self-injury.

Down Syndrome (DS)

Down syndrome (DS) is the most common chromosomal condition diagnosed in the USA and occurs in 1 out of every 700 children [17]. Down syndrome is often caused by having an extra chromosome 21. Individuals with DS usually have lower IQ than the general population and have some developmental delays.

- Facial characteristics associated with Down syndrome
  - Flatter face, with a flatter bridge of the nose
  - Upward-slanting, almond-shaped eyes
  - Shorter neck
  - Smaller ears
  - A tongue that protrudes from the mouth
  - Poorer muscle tone or joint laxity [18]
- Risk factors
  - Maternal age above 35 years
  - However, the majority of children with DS are born to mothers less than 35 years old
- Common co-occurring medical conditions
  - Hearing loss
  - Obstructive sleep apnea
  - Low vision including cataracts and severe refractive errors
  - Congenital heart defects
  - Neurologic dysfunction
  - Gastrointestinal atresia
  - Hip dislocation
  - Thyroid disease
  - Transient myeloproliferative disorder
  - Leukemia [19]

- Common co-occurring psychiatric conditions
  - Unlike other children with ID, children with DS are less likely to have maladaptive behaviors or emotional problems
  - ADHD was found to co-occur from 6% to 43%
  - Autism spectrum disorders in children with DS have been estimated to be ~5%
  - Depression
  - Delirium/dementia [20–23]
- *Clinical Pearl:* While individuals with Down syndrome may appear to be cheerful, it is important to keep in mind that each person has had differing life experiences, and their needs vary accordingly.

Williams Syndrome (WS)

Williams syndrome (WS) is a genetic disorder caused by a deletion from chromosome 7. It can result in mild-to-moderate ID, distinctive facial features, and some certain specific personality characteristics [24]. It occurs in approximately 1 in 10,000 births. Most cases of WS occur spontaneously

- Facial characteristics associated with Williams Syndrome include:
  - Broad forehead
  - Short nose with a broad tip
  - Full cheeks and wide mouth with full lips
- Personality characteristics associated with WS:
  - Friendly, sometimes described as "overly friendly"
  - Outgoing
  - Empathic [25, 26]
- Common co-occurring medical conditions:
  - Cardiac abnormalities
  - Dental irregularities
  - Hearing hypersensitivities [27]
- Common co-occurring psychiatric conditions:
  - Anxiety
  - ADHD
  - Depression [28]

- *Clinical Pearl*: Individuals with Williams syndrome are often outgoing and social, but they have a high co-occurrence of anxiety disorders.

Fragile X Syndrome

Fragile X syndrome (FXS) is caused by an expanding trinucleotide repeat on the X chromosome resulting in an individual, usually a man, developing the disorder.

- Common facial features include:
  - Large, protruding ears
  - Long face
  - High forehead
- Common co-occurring medical conditions:
  - Seizures
  - Recurrent otitis media and sinusitis
  - GERD
  - Women who carry the pre-mutation (trinucleotide repeat not meeting full FXS criteria) are at increased risk of premature ovarian failure [29]
- Common co-occurring psychiatric and behavioral conditions:
  - Autism-like behaviors—60% of males with FXS display behaviors that are frequent and severe enough to warrant a comorbid diagnosis of ASD
  - Intellectual disability
  - ADHD—hyperactivity, impulsivity, and inattention symptoms
  - Social anxiety
  - Unusual speech patterns and language delay [30]
- Treatment: Addressing co-occurring disorders and psycho-education for family and potential carriers.

Prader-Willi Syndrome

Most occurrences of Prader-Willi syndrome (PWS) are caused by the deletion of genes from chromosome 15. This causes certain syndrome-specific characteristics.

- Common features:
  - Poor feeding as an infant
  - During childhood, development of chronic overeating
  - Poor muscle tone
  - Poor growth and short stature
  - Delayed development and intellectual disabilities
- Common medical considerations in treatment of PWS:
  - Delayed puberty
  - Obesity
  - Epilepsy
  - Respiratory disorders
  - Central obstructive sleep apnea [31, 32]
- Psychiatric and behavioral symptoms in PWS:
  - Overeating—this symptom can be one of the most concerning to family and caregivers as this can be disruptive to a household. Management of diabetes mellitus can be challenging with this symptom as well.
  - Skin-picking—compulsive excoriation, or skin-picking, has been noted to occur more often in individuals with PWS.
  - Emotional outbursts or "tantrums"—unlike other genetic syndromes, individuals with PWS do not experience decreases in verbal aggression over time [33]
  - OCD-like symptoms
  - Autism-like symptoms
- Treatment:
  - To address "manipulative behaviors," firm limit-setting can be helpful as well as selective serotonin reuptake inhibitors (SSRIs) [33]
  - Polysomnogram for diagnosis of any sleep-related disorders
  - Healthy, moderate diet as best as can be managed
- *Clinical Pearl*: Individuals with PWS may have difficulty with communication and can benefit from limit-setting.

References

1. https://www.cdc.gov/ncbddd/fasd/diagnosis.html. Accessed 21 June 2018.
2. Lange S, et al. Global prevalence of fetal alcohol spectrum disorder among children and youth: a systematic review and meta-analysis. Obstet Gynecol Surv. 2018;73(4):189–91.
3. May PA, Phillip Gossage J. Maternal risk factors for fetal alcohol spectrum disorders: not as simple as it might seem. Alcohol Res Health. 2011;34(1):15.
4. Wilhoit LF, Scott DA, Simecka BA. Fetal alcohol spectrum disorders: characteristics, complications, and treatment. Community Ment Health J. 2017;53(6):711–8.
5. O'Connor MJ, et al. Psychiatric illness in a clinical sample of children with prenatal alcohol exposure. Am J Drug Alcohol Abuse. 2002;28(4):743–54.
6. Weyrauch D, et al. Comorbid mental disorders in fetal alcohol spectrum disorders: a systematic review. J Dev Behav Pediatr. 2017;38(4):283–91.
7. Silva D, et al. Comorbidities of attention deficit hyperactivity disorder: pregnancy risk factors and parent mental health. Community Ment Health J. 2015;51(6):738–45.
8. Streissguth AP, et al. Risk factors for adverse life outcomes in fetal alcohol syndrome and fetal alcohol effects. J Dev Behav Pediatr. 2004;25(4):228–38.
9. American Psychiatric Association. Diagnostic and statistical manual of mental disorders (DSM-5®). Arlington: American Psychiatric Pub; 2013.
10. https://www.cdc.gov/ncbddd/autism/data.html. Accessed 2018.
11. Wilkins J, Matson JL. A comparison of social skills profiles in intellectually disabled adults with and without ASD. Behav Modif. 2009;33(2):143–55.
12. Simonoff E, et al. Psychiatric disorders in children with autism spectrum disorders: prevalence, comorbidity, and associated factors in a population-derived sample. J Am Acad Child Adolesc Psychiatry. 2008;47(8):921–9.
13. Richards C, et al. Self-injurious behaviour in individuals with autism spectrum disorder and intellectual disability. J Intellect Disabil Res. 2012;56(5):476–89.

14. LeClerc S, Easley D. Pharmacological therapies for autism spectrum disorder: a review. P T. 2015;40(6):389.

15. Stehr-Green P, et al. Autism and thimerosal-containing vaccines: lack of consistent evidence for an association. Am J Prev Med. 2003;25(2):101–6.

16. Taylor LE, Swerdfeger AL, Eslick GD. Vaccines are not associated with autism: an evidence-based meta-analysis of case-control and cohort studies. Vaccine. 2014;32(29):3623–9.

17. Parker SE, et al. Updated national birth prevalence estimates for selected birth defects in the United States, 2004–2006. Birth Defects Res A Clin Mol Teratol. 2010;88(12):1008–16.

18. https://www.cdc.gov/ncbddd/birthdefects/DownSyndrome.html. Accessed 21 June 2018.

19. Bull MJ. Health supervision for children with Down syndrome. Am Acad Pediatr. 2011;128:393–406.

20. Dykens EM. Psychiatric and behavioral disorders in persons with down syndrome. Dev Disabil Res Rev. 2007;13(3):272–8.

21. DiGuiseppi C, et al. Screening for autism spectrum disorders in children with Down syndrome: population prevalence and screening test characteristics. J Dev Behav Pediatr. 2010;31(3):181.

22. Mantry D, et al. The prevalence and incidence of mental ill-health in adults with down syndrome. J Intellect Disabil Res. 2008;52(2):141–55.

23. Sivan E, et al. Down syndrome and attention-deficit/hyperactivity disorder (ADHD). J Child Neurol. 2011;26(10):1290–5.

24. https://ghr.nlm.nih.gov/condition/williams-syndrome. Accessed 21 June 2018.

25. Donnai D, Karmiloff-Smith A. Williams syndrome: from genotype through to the cognitive phenotype. Am J Med Genet A. 2000;97(2):164–71.

26. Dykens EM, Rosner BA. Refining behavioral phenotypes: personality—motivation in Williams and Prader-Willi syndromes. Am J Ment Retard. 1999;104(2):158–69.

27. Blomberg S, Rosander M, Andersson G. Fears, hyperacusis and musicality in Williams syndrome. Res Dev Disabil. 2006;27(6):668–80.

28. Leyfer OT, et al. Prevalence of psychiatric disorders in 4 to 16-year-olds with Williams syndrome. Am J Med Genet B Neuropsychiatr Genet. 2006;141(6):615–22.

29. Garber KB, Visootsak J, Warren ST. Fragile X syndrome. Eur J Hum Genet. 2008;16(6):666.

30. McDuffie A, et al. Symptoms of autism in males with fragile X syndrome: a comparison to nonsyndromic ASD using current ADI-R scores. J Autism Dev Disord. 2015;45(7):1925–37.
31. Thomson AK, Glasson EJ, Bittles AH. A long-term population-based clinical and morbidity review of Prader–Willi syndrome in Western Australia. J Intellect Disabil Res. 2006;50(1):69–78.
32. Festen DAM, et al. Sleep-related breathing disorders in pre-pubertal children with Prader-Willi syndrome and effects of growth hormone treatment. J Clin Endocrinol Metabol. 2006;91(12):4911–5.
33. Rice LJ, et al. The developmental trajectory of disruptive behavior in Down syndrome, fragile X syndrome, Prader–Willi syndrome and Williams syndrome. Am J Med Genet C Semin Med Genet. 2015;169(2):182–7.

Chapter 16
Trauma- and Stressor- Related Disorders

David W. Dixon

Factors and Predisposition

- People with ID, like the general population, will be exposed to stress throughout their lives. When stress becomes overwhelming or experiences rise to the level of trauma, psychopathological symptoms can emerge.
- The timing and type of trauma or stress combined with the response, developmental age, previous experiences, environment, and biopsychosocial factors will all play roles in determining symptomatology and outcomes for patients.
- People with ID are more likely to have experienced trauma during developmental years that may affect their ability to navigate healthy relationships with secure attachments.
- Individuals with ID may reach the threshold for clinically significant trauma- and stressor- related disorders with less serious events than are required for the general population.

D. W. Dixon (✉)
San Antonio Military Medical Center, Houston, TX, USA
e-mail: david.dixon@wright.edu

© Springer Nature Switzerland AG 2019
J. P. Gentile et al. (eds.), *Guide to Intellectual Disabilities*,
https://doi.org/10.1007/978-3-030-04456-5_16

Evaluation

General Guidelines

- Ruling out medical conditions should be the first step to any evaluation of mental disturbance.
- Individuals with ID may develop symptoms that look like depression/anxiety/trauma responses from a wide array of medical problems [1, 2].
  - Reflux disease, migraines, substance/medication side effects/withdrawals, infections (urinary tract, ear, or cellulitis), pain, constipation, thyroid abnormalities, obstructive sleep apnea, dementia, delirium, or catatonia can present with symptoms that mimic trauma.
- Sudden onset of severe symptoms warrants thorough medical evaluation.
- A thorough history obtained from caregivers and the patient is crucial.
- Use developmentally appropriate language when directly questioning the patient (e.g., "Are you feeling happy?")
- For patients with limited verbal communication skills, or limited cognitive abilities, use yes/no or closed questions to screen [2]. Limit the use of open-ended questions to clarify specific points or when talking with caregivers or family. Limiting conversation to concrete rather than abstract topics may be higher yield when interviewing the individual.
- Utilization of visual scales or asking about mood changes (e.g., feelings of sadness) should be performed in conjunction with an observation of affect by the provider [3].
- Information from caregivers and family should be as objective as possible with specific behaviors identified and with careful attention given to acute changes.
- Establish a clear picture of the baseline routine and function for the patient. Discuss this at every visit to identify insidious changes not directly observable by staff with daily interaction.
- Psychosocial factors can have profound effects and often compound mental health symptoms.

- Develop a timeline and the course of symptoms from care-givers if patients are unable to be specific (consider using recent anchor events/holidays to establish a timeline from patients).
- Ask about the time frame surrounding symptoms; try to identify any changes to routine, living conditions, social involvement, occupational changes, family members, stressors, or trauma.

Adjustment Disorder/Posttraumatic Stress Disorder/Acute Stressor Disorder

- Establish whether the patient has been exposed to a trauma or stressor which could be contributing to present-ing symptoms.
- Consider that people with ID may experience high levels of stress (which becomes traumatic) from situations that may otherwise be a normal part of life [3], such as:
  - Moving
  - Favorite staff member receiving promotion and transi-tioning to a new position (resulting in decreased inter-face with patient)
  - Romantic breakup
  - Consensual sexual experiences
- Patients may develop repetitive memories or flashbacks of trauma that are disruptive.
  - Caregivers of patients with severe/profound ID may observe the patient acting out the traumatic events or self-injuring in response to memories of trauma [3].
- Establish an understanding of patient sleeping patterns, habits, behaviors, and environment (e.g., bedtime, waking time, nocturnal waking, naps, quality of sleep, nightmares/dreams, snoring, screens/sounds in room, temperature fluc-tuations, type of bedding, or roommates.)
- Discuss with the patient whether they are experiencing nightmares. If so, try to establish whether the content or emotions of dreams might be related to the trauma. Patients with significant cognitive impairments may not be able to share the content of dreams.

- If possible, try to quantify how often dreams are occurring (e.g., twice a week or every night), which can be helpful data to have when evaluating efficacy of treatment.
- Individuals with ID may also present with disorganization or agitation whenever they are reminded of their traumatic experiences and will often take steps to keep distant from such reminders (e.g., caregivers reporting noncompliance with usual activities).
  - The lower the developmental age, the lower the threshold for reminders to be causes of stress reaction in individuals with ID.
- When patients are having a difficult time recalling parts of their trauma, assess whether this is a result of their baseline functioning, a reaction to the trauma, or the result of a substance or physical symptom related to the trauma (e.g., TBI, ingestion of substances during the event, or loss of consciousness).
- Discuss with patient and caregivers whether the patient has been demonstrating a change in their interest in other people or favorite activities, more sadness, or a more pessimistic view on their lives.
  - Take into consideration that some patients may not hold positive views of the future without any exposure to trauma (e.g., "I won't be able to drive." "I won't have children." "I won't get married.")
- Evaluate for decreased concentration that may be observed by acute changes in the ability to work or play, intermittent difficulties with memory, or difficulty completing common tasks [3].
- Other symptoms to be aware of may include clinging to caregivers, loss of skills, withdrawal, irritability, aggression, enhanced sensory sensitivity, or anger.
- Timelines and severity of symptoms may be helpful with diagnosis:
  - PTSD and acute stress disorder will present with more severe symptoms.
  - PTSD and adjustment disorder may be present for longer periods of time.
  - Adjustment disorder may present with milder symptoms.

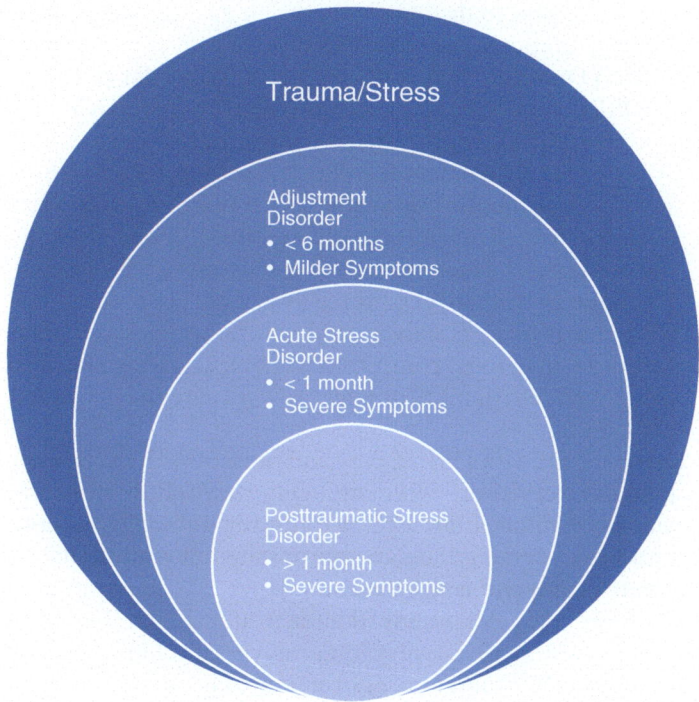

Reactive Attachment Disorder/Disinhibited Social Engagement Disorder

- Patients with reactive attach ment disorder (RAD) and disinhibited social engagement disorder (DSED) will present with very different primary symptoms [4–6]:
  - RAD with withdrawal from others.
  - DSED with carefree familiarity with strangers.
- However, in each of these conditions, there is a history of traumatic upbringing during the early developmental stages of life [5].
- When a patient is suspected of suffering from one of these diagnoses, a thorough evaluation of their early upbringing

can be helpful to distinguish between disorders with similar presentations:
- RAD may look like autism spectrum disorder or PTSD.
- DSED may look like attention deficit hyperactivity disorder, PTSD, or poor social judgment.

- A history of living in an institutional setting, foster care, or with emotionally unavailable/withholding/constantly changing caregivers in the early months of life may signify the presence of a lack of secure attachments for the patient.
- For patients with RAD, they will present with emotional withdrawal from caregivers and will rarely seek out comfort or be able to be comforted when upset. They may also present with irritability or anger toward caregivers without explanation [4].
- For patients with DSED, they will present with excessively casual interactions with strangers, have little restraint when communicating with or following unfamiliar people, and fail to demonstrate an appropriate amount of anxiety when a caregiver is not around [5].
- Patients with ASD may demonstrate similar levels of withdrawal or disinterest in caregivers, though a history of neglectful/traumatic upbringing may or may not be present.
- Consider the patient's developmental age and compare to patients with similar disabilities/developmental age before making a diagnosis.
- Always consider the possibility of co-morbid diagnoses that may affect the course and severity of illness like depression, anxiety, PTSD, or ADHD.

Treatment

General Considerations

- If the abuse or trauma is ongoing, remove the patient from the situation and report as required by local, state, or federal regulations.

- The use of benzodiazepines in the ID population is recommended only with extra caution due to increased risk of disinhibition, worsened self-injurious behaviors, hyperactivity, or withdrawal-induced manic symptoms.
- When behavioral concerns are present, consult behavioral support specialists.
- Consider music or art therapy consultation.
- Do not assume that individuals with ID are not sexually active and will not/cannot become pregnant.

Adjustment Disorder/Posttraumatic Stress Disorder/Acute Stress Disorder

- Psychotherapy should be considered first-line treatment.
- Eye movement and desensitization processing (EMDR) therapy has been demonstrated in small studies to be beneficial to reduce symptoms with gains lasting as long as 2.5 years.
- Psychotherapeutic interventions are effective but may require modification to address decreased verbal, expressive, or cognitive abilities.
- Treatment should be catered to the patient's specific needs.
- See Chap. 11 for more information on adapted therapies.
- SSRIs and SNRIs are appropriate to manage depressive/anxious symptoms.
- α1-antagonists (e.g., prazosin) may prove useful when titrated slowly to manage nightmare or hyperarousal symptoms.
  - Twice-daily dosing may improve daytime hyperarousal symptoms.
- Benzodiazepines should be avoided if possible.
- Medications should be chosen based on symptoms. Comorbid conditions such as hypothyroidism, attention deficit hyperactivity disorder, or cardiac disease should also be considered when choosing a medication. Risk factors for potential side effects should be evaluated. Care should be taken to monitor for adverse effects that may be more

likely in this population like the higher rates of epilepsy that could limit the use of bupropion.

- See Chap. 10 for further details on antidepressant and α1-antagonist medications.
- Titrate the medication based on clinical presentation rather than prescribing standard doses.
- The patient should be frequently evaluated for adverse effects, side effects, efficacy of treatment, response, or remission.
- Patients should have medications titrated and tapered under careful observation, and side effects should be preferentially managed by subtracting causative medications rather than adding new medications.

Reactive Attachment Disorder/Disinhibited Social Engagement Disorder (See Table 16.1)

- The focus for treatment of either disorder should be placed on establishing healthy attachments for the patient.
- Consistent, attentive, and caring figures are vital and should be clearly established for the patient.
- Psychotherapy can be beneficial as well. Patients should be linked with therapists who have demonstrated proficiency in managing these disorders.
- There are no psychopharmacologic recommendations for RAD or DSED; however, treatment of co-morbid or underlying mental health conditions may require the use of medications.

Conclusion

- Patients with ID may present with symptoms of reactivity to trauma after experiencing stressors that may not be expected to cause such reactions.
- Taking time to understand the etiology of a patient's symptoms can help in the diagnosis and treatment of trauma-related disorders.

TABLE 16.1 Adapted Criteria for Reactive Detachment Disorder and Disinhibited Social Engagement Disorder (adapted from DM-ID, Second Edition)

Reactive attachment disorder (criteria with *adaptations* from DM-ID-2)	Disinhibited social engagement disorder (criteria with *adaptations* from DM-ID-2)
The patient is >9 months (developmentally)	*The patient is >9 months (developmentally)*
With one of the following (historically):	*With one of the following (historically):*
A pattern of emotional abandonment or withholding of warmth, solace, or excitation from caregivers (*no adaptation*)	A pattern of emotional abandonment or withholding of warmth, solace, or excitation from caregivers (*no adaptation*)
A pattern of transitioning caregivers without ability to successfully develop stable attachments (*no adaptation*)	A pattern of transitioning caregivers without ability to successfully develop stable attachments (*no adaptation*)
Upbringing in settings that provided limited circumstances to form selective attachments (*no adaptation*)	Upbringing in settings that provided limited circumstances to form selective attachments (*no adaptation*)
Resulting in both of the following:	*Resulting in at least two of the following:*
The patient does not typically look for consolation *in a developmentally appropriate fashion, or may exhibit agitated, impaired, or aggressive behaviors with distress*	*When compared to children of similar measured intelligence, adaptive skills, or sensory impairments,* little to no restraint while communicating with unknown people
The patient has inappropriately mild relief with attempts at consolation *including refusing comforting or becoming agitated, aggressive, or destructive with comforting in a maladaptive way*	Excessively casual interactions that exceeds the age-, culturally, socially, *or developmentally appropriate* norms

(continued)

TABLE 16.1 (continued)

Reactive attachment disorder (criteria with *adaptations* from DM-ID-2)	Disinhibited social engagement disorder (criteria with *adaptations* from DM-ID-2)
	A reduction, or failure, to seek the approval of a caregiver before wandering away in an unknown setting (*no adaptation*)
	An inclination to accompany a stranger with little, or no, pause *that is not due to lapses in judgment due to cognitive, emotional, or adaptive deficits*
As well as two of the following:	*Symptoms are independent of the impulsivity from ADHD*
Limited reaction, emotionally or socially, to those around them (*no adaptation*)	
Decreased ability to demonstrate good moods *despite appropriate environmental setting for adaptive functioning and positive support*	
Occasional events highlighted by irascibility, negative mood, or anxiousness even while being supported by caregivers – *not during times of transition or with traumatic reminders*	
Symptoms started before patient turned 5 years old	
Does *not* have autism spectrum disorder *or behaviors are distinct from autism spectrum disorder*	

TABLE 16.1 (continued)

Reactive attachment disorder (criteria with *adaptations* from DM-ID-2)	Disinhibited social engagement disorder (criteria with *adaptations* from DM-ID-2)
Reactive attachment disorder	Disinhibited social engagement disorder
The patient is > 9 months (developmentally)	*The patient is > 9 months (developmentally)*
With one of the following (historically):	*With one of the following (historically):*
A pattern of emotional abandonment or withholding of warmth, solace, or excitation from caregivers (*no adaptation*)	A pattern of emotional abandonment or withholding of warmth, solace, or excitation from caregivers (*no adaptation*)
A pattern of transitioning caregivers without ability to successfully develop stable attachments (*no adaptation*)	A pattern of transitioning caregivers without ability to successfully develop stable attachments (*no adaptation*)
Upbringing in settings that provided limited circumstances to form selective attachments (*no adaptation*)	Upbringing in settings that provided limited circumstances to form selective attachments (*no adaptation*)
Resulting in both of the following:	*Resulting in at least two of the following:*
The patient does not typically look for consolation *in a developmentally appropriate fashion, or may exhibit agitated, impaired, or aggressive behaviors with distress*	*When compared to children of similar measured intelligence, adaptive skills, or sensory impairments,* little to no restraint while communicating with unknown people
The patient has inappropriately mild relief with attempts at consolation *including refusing comforting or becoming agitated, aggressive, or destructive with comforting in a maladaptive way*	Excessively casual interactions that exceeds the age-, culturally, socially, *or developmentally appropriate* norms

(continued)

Table 16.1 (continued)

Reactive attachment disorder (criteria with *adaptations* from DM-ID-2)	Disinhibited social engagement disorder (criteria with *adaptations* from DM-ID-2)
	A reduction, or failure, to seek the approval of a caregiver before wandering away in an unknown setting (*no adaptation*)
As well as two of the following:	An inclination to accompany a stranger with little, or no, pause *that is not due to lapses in judgment due to cognitive, emotional, or adaptive deficits Symptoms are independent of the impulsivity from ADHD*
Limited reaction, emotionally or socially, to those around them (*no adaptation*) Decreased ability to demonstrate good moods *despite appropriate environmental setting for adaptive functioning and positive support* Occasional events highlighted by irascibility, negative mood, or anxiousness even while being supported by caregivers – *not during times of transition or with traumatic reminders* Symptoms started before patient turned 5 years old Does *not* have autism spectrum disorder *or behaviors are distinct from autism spectrum disorder*	

- Taking the patient's developmental age will assist in identifying and treating RAD and DSED.
- Psychotherapy can, and should, be utilized in the treatment of trauma- and stressor-related disorders in the ID population.

Clinical Pearls
- Trauma and social stressors can often mimic other psychiatric disorders, especially psychotic disorders
- Obtain a trauma and attachment history to have a thorough understanding of the individual with ID
- Appropriate treatment of trauma- and stressor-related disorders is often psychotherapy. Medications are sometimes indicated

References

1. Fletcher RJ, Barnhill J, Cooper SA. DM-ID-2: diagnostic manual-intellectual disability: a textbook of diagnosis of mental disorders in persons with intellectual disability. Washington, D.C.: National Assn for the Dually Diagnosed Press; 2016.
2. Gentile JP, Gillig PM, editors. Psychiatry of intellectual disability: a practical manual. Hoboken: John Wiley & Sons; 2012.
3. Mevissen L, et al. Treatment of PTSD in people with severe intellectual disabilities; a case series. Dev Neurorehabil. 2012;15(3):223–32.
4. Minnis H, Fleming G, Cooper S. Reactive attachment disorder symptoms in adults with intellectual disabilities. J Appl Res Intellect Disabil. 2010;23:398–403.
5. Van Ijzendoorn MH, Scheungel C, Bakermans-Kranenburg Mj. Disorganized attachment in early childhood: meta-analysis of precursors, comcomitants & sequelae. Dev Psychol. 1999;11:225–49.
6. Zeanah C, et al. Practice parameter for the assessment and treatment of children and adolescents with reactive attachment disorder and disinhibited social engagement disorder. J Am Acad Child Adolesc Psychiatry. 2016;55(11):990–1003.

Chapter 17
Personality Disorders

Allison E. Cowan

The diagnosis of personality disorders in persons with intellectual disability (ID) remains controversial [1]. Data regarding prevalence likewise is wide ranging [2]. One study in older adults with ID showed increased odds for diagnosis of personality disorder [3], but there continues to be a gap in the literature. The DM-ID-2 (2016) cautions mental health professionals to remain aware of the cultural background in which many individuals with ID were raised. The authors describe the "twin traps of, on the one hand, declaring that individuals with IDD are immune from some personality disorders or, on the other hand, suggesting that these individuals present in ways grossly divergent from individuals without IDD" [4]. Table 17.1 describes some common issues in co-occurring personality disorder and intellectual disability (Table 17.1).

A. E. Cowan (✉)
Department of Psychiatry, Wright State University,
Dayton, OH, USA
e-mail: Allison.cowan@wright.edu

© Springer Nature Switzerland AG 2019
J. P. Gentile et al. (eds.), *Guide to Intellectual Disabilities*,
https://doi.org/10.1007/978-3-030-04456-5_17

TABLE 17.1 Issues related to personality disorder diagnosis in individuals with ID from DM-ID-2

Individuals with ID are likely to experience a delayed development that may result in an immature or a less completely developed personality, since the DSM-5 places emphasis on what is culturally acceptable.

Difficulty with empathy should be considered in the context of the individuals with ID as development of this ability to imagine the perspective of another represents a developmental milestone.

Individuals with previous experience in institutional settings could have adapted to institutional life by developing behavioral and cognitive patterns that are consistent with personality disorder.

DM-ID-2 authors suggest that individuals with severe or profound ID do not have sufficiently developed personality disorders that a reliable diagnosis of personality disorder can be made.

Making the Diagnosis

- The Royal College of Psychiatrists suggest key points regarding personality disorders:
  - A higher age threshold (over 23 years) is advised for diagnosing personality disorders.
  - The categories of schizoid, dependent, and anxious/avoidant personality disorders are not recommended.
  - Initial diagnosis using the criteria for personality disorder—Unspecified—is suggested [5].
- Personality disorders are described as an "enduring patter of inner experience and behavior that deviates markedly from the expectations of the individual's culture, is pervasive and inflexible, has an onset in adolescence or early adulthood, is stable over time, and leads to distress or impairment" [6].

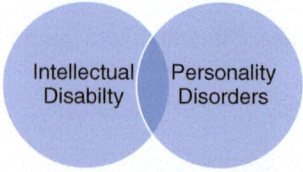

Treatment of Personality Disorders

- The most common treatment for personality disorders is regular psychotherapy.
- Occasionally, medications may be prescribed to target specific symptoms, but psychotherapy is considered better at treating the core symptoms of personality disorders.
- Certain therapies are tailored to specific disorders and some have been further modified for use in persons with ID. Cognitive behavioral therapy, dialectical behavioral therapy, supportive therapy, and psychodynamic psychotherapy have been adapted for use in persons with ID. Dialectical behavioral therapy has been adapted for use in ID and borderline personality.

Paranoid Personality Disorder

Paranoid personality disorder is characterized by pervasive distrust and suspiciousness of others. Individuals with paranoid personality disorder often interpret the actions of other people as being exploitative, harmful, or deceptive [6].

- There remains minimal evidence about the co-occurrence of paranoid personality disorder in individuals with ID, but a community survey of 101 individuals with ID found 5 met criteria for the diagnosis [7]. This is close to 5%, which is higher than other studies of the population as a whole.
- People with ID are at higher risk for exploitation and deception. It is also likely they have been taken advantage of in the past. It is necessary to remember that current suspicions may, in fact, be true.
- The DM-ID-2 notes that some of the diagnostic criteria requires a "considerable degree of abstract thinking and ability to understand things in perspective" and that this may impact presentation of individuals with ID [4]. Misunderstandings, or sometimes too commonly, caregivers not explaining situations in easily understood ways can impact this criterion.

- The anger that can accompany this disorder should be considered in the context of ID, which is that with limited means of coping and limited personal control over many things, anger may result.
- Worry of a romantic partner cheating on the patient can be a reasonable suspicion and fear. The speed at which people initiate and then end relationships at supported employment settings should also be taken into consideration. Additionally, the smaller available dating pool should also be considered.

Schizoid Personality Disorder

Schizoid personality disorder is described as a pattern of disinterest and detachment from social interactions [6]. The Diagnostic Criteria for Learning Disabilities suggests not using this diagnosis for individuals with ID [5]. Many of the diagnostic criteria are dependent on the individual's ability to communicate fairly abstract and difficult-to-convey inner states of being.

- Because opportunity of socialization often does not depend on the desires of the individual with ID, determining whether someone prefers to be alone is crucial.
- People with ID may have learned not to expect social outings because of repeated disappointments with practical barriers like the functionality of caregivers' cars, money, or the ability of the other individual to spend time together.
- Those with ID have increased supervision and are frequently discouraged from expressing sexual thoughts and feeling that are depicted as "inappropriate." There is also widespread cultural stigma regarding the discussion of sexual topics.
- Individuals with ID are often given a significantly limited selection of activities to participate in and are often limited by the activities that caregivers choose.
- Social circles of patients with ID are often limited due to logistical constraints rather than desire.

- Genetic syndromes, medication, and differing brain structures can impact how emotions are conveyed and affect/emotional expression can be limited.

Schizotypal Personality Disorder

Schizotypal personality disorder is characterized by limited interest and deficits in interpersonal interaction as well as other eccentricities of thought. There again is limited information about individuals with co-occurring ID and schizotypal personality disorder. The DM-ID-2 cautions that many of the criteria involved are styles of thinking and also encourages the clinician to be aware of the client group as a whole and to consider these characteristics in relation to cultural patterns that are acceptable among peers who have ID [4].

- In individuals with ID, ideas of reference should be differentiated from delusions of reference and from wishful thinking.
- Some individuals with ID believe they are police and officers, firefighters, security guards, and workshop supervisors. They will even have paraphernalia consistent with these beliefs—lanyards with named tags, badges, and safety vests. This is typically culturally accepted in the ID community.
- In considering speech style, many individuals with ID have idiosyncrasies in speech due to expressive language barriers and limited vocabularies.
- When considering if a patient with ID is overly suspicious of others, remember that they are at increased risk for exploitation.
- Unusual or childlike interests are common in the ID population and should be kept in mind when considering this criterion.
- Persons with ID frequently have external restrictions on socializing, so it may be difficult to discern lack of interest with lack of opportunity.

Antisocial Personality Disorder

Antisocial personality disorder is described as a pervasive pattern of disregard for and violation of the rights of others, occurring since childhood [6]. Much of the information about ID and antisocial personality comes from studies of offender populations. Upwards of 40% of incarcerated people with ID were found to have antisocial personality disorder [1]. In a self-reported study on antisocial behavior, a significantly higher prevalence of such behavior was reported in the ID sample, but the authors suggest that higher rates of social deprivation and mental illness accounted for these differences [8].

- A certain disregard for laws, right and wrong, and morality is integral to antisocial personality disorder.
  - If an individual understands laws and the difference between right and wrong, this diagnosis should be considered. If, however, they do not have the abstract cognitive skills for this understanding, antisocial personality disorder may not be the appropriate diagnosis.
- The cognitive ability of the patient should also be considered when making this diagnosis. Planning ahead to take advantage of others requires a fairly significant amount of cognitive skills, which may be difficult to meet for individuals with moderate ID, and likely not possible for those with severe-profound ID.
- Anger and temper are both a feature of this disorder as well as a feature of ID. Care should be taken to examine the situation where an individual is aggressive with the appropriate use of behavioral analysis to determine causative events.
- While a substandard employment history can be a feature of antisocial personality disorder, employment is not always left to the discretion of the person with ID. The job, supervisor, and workshop call all be assigned positions.
- The DM-ID-2 notes that the "suitability of [lack of remorse] requires that the individual has a well-developed ability to understand things in perspective, allowing him or

her to understand the feelings of others and to regret actions. Such an ability becomes increasingly unlikely in individuals with increasing severities of IDD" [4].

- Additionally, there are often many people on a treatment team. There can be repetition of conversations with multiple members of the team that can be emotionally fatiguing. Lack of remorse should be supported by evidence from a collateral source with whom the individual in question has a good relationship.
- The DM-ID-2 recommends 21 years of age and evidence of conduct disorder before age 18 [4].

Borderline Personality Disorder

Borderline personality disorder is characterized by emotionality, disturbances in mood, impulsivity, and impairments in interpersonal relationships. There remains a lack of literature about the co-occurrence of ID and borderline personality, but there can be significant overlapping in symptoms.

- The concerns about abandonment that can be a core feature of borderline personality disorder is also a feature of living with ID. The DM-ID-2 notes that persons with ID are reliant on caregivers more than individuals without ID [4]. A caregiver not showing up for a shift or a parent not being on time might represent a real emergency with lack of access to meals and transportation. There are regular staffing turnovers at sheltered workshops and group homes that, if recognized, can be addressed in compassionate terms with regard to grief and loss but, if unaddressed, could present similarly to borderline personality disorder.
- Individuals with ID can have limited coping skills and impaired cognitive abilities that can lead to difficulties with overlapping borderline personality disorder symptoms.
  - Spending money without concern for practicalities
  - Anger outbursts

- Difficulty waiting
- Self-injury when upset or in pain
- Treatment of individuals with ID and borderline personality disorder requires the solidarity of the team and understanding how best to help the patient.
  - Frequent team meetings are helpful in handling team splitting.
  - Dialectical behavioral therapy has been adapted for use in individuals with ID and borderline personality.
  - While polypharmacy is often seen in both patients with ID as well as those with borderline personality disorder, it is discouraged.

Histrionic Personality Disorder

Histrionic personality disorder is described as a pattern of excessive, shallow emotionality and attention seeking [6]. The DM-ID-2 suggests that the symptoms count needed for diagnosis be reduced from five to four out of six due to lack of applicability to individuals with ID [4]. Additionally, this diagnosis was considered for exclusion in DSM-5 because of a lack of evidence of scientific validity.

- Individuals with ID are sometimes accused of being "attention seeking" as though all people do not need interaction with others. Remember that seeking out interactions with others when a person has communication and cognitive limitations can be different than those without ID.
- Individuals with ID and co-occurring histrionic personality disorder may interrupt others and want to be in others' conversations, or they may have limited social skills.
- Some common descriptors of both individuals with ID and those with histrionic personality disorder are:
  - Unusual appearance
  - Speaking unclearly or struggling with conveying details
  - Emotional

- If a person with ID is presenting with overly sexualized conversations or actions, they should be screened for sexual abuse or exploitation.

Narcissistic Personality Disorder

Narcissistic personality disorder is characterized by a pattern of grandiose thinking or behavior, need for admiration, and lack of empathy [6]. Because many of the criteria of this disorder are dependent on both expressive language skills and the lack of progression through normal development to produce things like humility and empathy, this diagnosis should be considered cautiously and only with reliable collateral history.

- Individuals with ID can have inflated sense of importance, and the authors of the DM-ID-2 suggest that if this is over and beyond what is considered culturally acceptable in persons with ID, narcissistic personality disorder can be considered [4].
  - Narcissism about being "the best helper" or "the fastest runner" is likely a culturally appropriate statement from an individual with ID.
- Commonalities to the diagnoses of ID and narcissistic personality disorder are:
  - Believing oneself is "special"
  - Believing oneself is the center of the family and that needs should be met quickly
  - Limited ability to empathize—these may derive from different etiologies but may present similarly

Avoidant Personality Disorder

Avoidant personality disorder is described as a pervasive pattern of social inhibition, feelings of inadequacy, and hypersensitivity to negative evaluation, beginning by early adulthood and present in a variety of contexts [6]. There are no adaptations to the criteria for avoidant personality disorder in the DM-ID-2, but they do note that individuals with ID may be more unwilling to become involved with others for reasonable fears of criticism and repeated failure [4]. Additionally, people with ID may be more likely to heed the advice of caregivers that strangers can be dangerous and that the world is full of potential danger.

Dependent Personality Disorder

Given that the nature of ID is to be more dependent on others for financial decisions, for menu planning, for work placement, and for many other parts of life, the diagnosis of dependent personality disorder is likely not a valid diagnosis for individuals with ID. Because being dependent on others is an adaptive trait with individuals and the diagnosis of a disorder in the DSM-5 requires impairment of functioning, this diagnosis does not fit this patient population.

Obsessive-Compulsive Personality Disorder

Obsessive-compulsive personality disorder (OCDP) is described as a pervasive pattern of preoccupation with orderliness, perfectionism, and mental and interpersonal control, at the expense of flexibility, openness, and efficiency [6]. Many features of this personality disorder have significant overlap with not only autism spectrum disorders (ASD) but with obsessive-compulsive disorder (OCD).

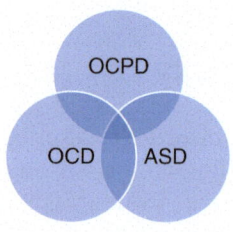

- Similarities between autism spectrum disorders and OCPD
  - Rigidity and inflexibility
  - Preoccupation with details or parts of things
  - Needing things to be done "just so"
  - Devotion to work
    - Individuals with ID often socialize at work, so dedication to workshop attendance and productivity must be considered in this regard.
- Similarities between OCPD and OCD
  - Hoarding behavior
    - Individuals with ID who have had institutional placements will often struggle with discarding these items.
    - Sentimentality can require a higher level of expressive communication than possible for some patients with ID, which can mean that items are meaningful, but caregivers are unable to discern the meaning.
  - Needing things to be done in a very specific manner
- Treatment of these disorders varies a great deal, which makes accurate diagnosis important.
  - OCPD is treated primarily with psychotherapy with focusing on being able to tolerate emotional closeness and easing of the unnecessarily strict rules.
  - ASD is treated with behavioral interventions, occupational therapy, sensory integration therapy, and occasionally medications when needed.
  - OCD is typically treated with a combination of medications and psychotherapy.

Conclusion

Diagnosing personality disorders in individuals with ID remains controversial. Guidance can be found in the work of the DM-ID-2 and the DSM-5. When diagnosing these disorders, it is imperative to consider the cultural context of ID and what is considered acceptable and developmentally appropriate, reliable collateral information as well as thorough screening for other psychiatric and medical disorders.

Clinical Pearls
- Treatment of personality disorders is primarily via psychotherapy rather than medications.
- Patients with ID live in a culture where certain things are acceptable that would not be in individuals without ID like being dependent on others.
- Anger and self-injury are common among the ID population and are not necessarily part of a personality disorder unless there are other supporting criteria present across many contexts.
- There is significant overlap between ID itself and personality disorders, so care should be taken in making the diagnosis.

Do's and Don't's

Do assess for personality disorders	Don't forget to account for the culture of ID
Do consider borderline personality disorder	Don't confuse self-injury of another etiology, e.g., pain, stimming, communication barriers
Do treat personality disorders with psychotherapy	Don't (or try not to) treat personality disorders primarily with medications

References

1. Lindsay WR, et al. Two studies on the prevalence and validity of personality disorder in three forensic intellectual disability samples. J Forensic Psychiatry Psychol. 2006;17(3):485–506.
2. Deb S, Thomas M, Bright C. Mental disorder in adults with intellectual disability. 1: prevalence of functional psychiatric illness among a community-based population aged between 16 and 64 years. J Intellect Disabil Res. 2001;45(6):495–505.
3. Axmon A, et al. Psychiatric diagnoses in older people with intellectual disability in comparison with the general population: a register study. Epidemiol Psychiatr Sci. 2018;27(5):479–91.

4. Fletcher RJ, Barnhill J, Cooper SA. DM-ID-2: diagnostic manual-intellectual disability: a textbook of diagnosis of mental disorders in persons with intellectual disability. Kingston: National Assn for the Dually Diagnosed Press; 2016.
5. Royal College of Psychiatrists. DC-LD: diagnostic criteria for psychiatric disorders for use with adults with learning disabilities/mental retardation, Vol. 48. London: Springer Science & Business; 2001.
6. American Psychiatric Association. Diagnostic and statistical manual of mental disorders (DSM-5®). Washington, DC: American Psychiatric Pub; 2013.
7. Khan A, Cowan C, Roy A. Personality disorders in people with learning disabilities: a community survey. J Intellect Disabil Res. 1997;41(4):324–30.
8. Dickson K, Emerson E, Hatton C. Self-reported anti-social behaviour: prevalence and risk factors amongst adolescents with and without intellectual disability. J Intellect Disabil Res. 2005;49(11):820–6.

Index

© Springer Nature Switzerland AG 2019
J. P. Gentile et al. (eds.), *Guide to Intellectual Disabilities*,
https://doi.org/10.1007/978-3-030-04456-5

The manufacturer's authorised representative in the EU is Springer
Nature Customer Service Centre GmbH, Europaplatz 3, 69115 Heidelberg,
Germany. If you have any concerns regarding our products, please
contact ProductSafety@springernature.com

Printed and bound by CPI Group (UK) Ltd, Croydon, CR0 4YY
29/04/2026
02099451-0001